T0199535

A Country Doctor in the French Revolution

This book will be of interest to those studying French medical and Revolutionary history. It traces the life of an early-modern rural French physician from childhood to death – how he worked as a physician for six years in North Africa (taking a particular interest in medical meteorology); sought to establish himself as a savant in the Republic of Letters by publishing texts and prize-winning essays; and, despite his bourgeois roots, took part in the siege of Toulon, became committed to the ideals of the French Revolution, and volunteered for the Revolutionary armée d'Italie, mainly working in military hospitals. It concludes with an account of his time practising medicine in southwest France, where he also engaged in local politics, eventually being appointed to a mayoral position by Bonaparte.

Robert Weston is Honorary Research Fellow at the University of Western Australia.

A Country Doctor in the French Revolution

Marie-François-Bernadin Ramel

Robert Weston

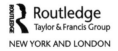
Routledge
Taylor & Francis Group

NEW YORK AND LONDON

First published 2020
by Routledge
52 Vanderbilt Avenue, New York, NY 10017

and by Routledge
2 Park Square, Milton Park, Abingdon, Oxon, OX14 4RN

Routledge is an imprint of the Taylor & Francis Group, an informa business

© 2020 Taylor & Francis

Library of Congress Cataloging-in-Publication Data
A catalog record for this title has been requested

ISBN: 978-0-367-27189-3 (hbk)
ISBN: 978-0-429-29539-3 (ebk)

Typeset in Times New Roman
by codeMantra

Contents

Figures

Tables

Notes on the Text

There are some apparent discrepancies in the archives over the dates attributed to events. I have recorded these as they appear in the records and, where significant, commented on the anomalies. Translations from French are my own. The orthography of eighteenth-century France was often different from that of today; when quoting material from that period the original orthography has been retained. The period covered by this study was one in which medicine was taught and practised based on theories which had been followed for centuries.

Acknowledgements

The input of many individuals is gratefully acknowledged. The archivists of Bibliothèque de l'Academie Nationale de Médicine, Paris; Bibliothèque interuniversitair de santé, Paris; les archives municipal de La Ciotat; les archives municipal d'Aubagne; les archives de la Chambre de commerce et d'industrie de Marseille-Provence; Ministère de la Défense, service historique de la défense centre historique des archives, Vincennes; Professor Susan Broomhall for reading earlier versions of this text and whose suggestions have improved the work; the anonymous reviewers whose helpful criticisms have polished the whole; and my wife Jan for her patience whilst this project has seemed as though it would never be completed.

1 Introduction

This book examines the life of an early-modern French physician, Marie-François-Bernadin Ramel le fils, who lived in the Marseille region. What makes this man of particular interest is the unusual pattern of his career, including working in North Africa, his activities during the French revolution, his responses to the subsequent social milieu, and his successes in contributing to the Republic of Medicine. There were thousands of doctors working in the smaller towns and villages in early-modern France, but few left a mark on the social and medical history of the period. It is unusual to find a rural physician such as Ramel to leave as remarkable a story as he did.

Structurally, I have largely worked chronologically through the life of Ramel. Needless to say, such an approach does not work perfectly. Chapter 2 examines Ramel's family background and Ramel's early education in Aubagne, a small French country town and Marseille. After completing a medical degree at Aix-en-Provence, Ramel travelled to North Africa; Chapter 3 is concerned with the six years he spent there, working in the local hospital and taking meteorological readings. Chapter 4 opens with his return to mainland France practising medicine. Ramel's efforts to establish himself as a *savant* in the Republic of Medicine are detailed in Chapter 5. The next two chapters address Ramel's involvement with the French Revolution and in particular his experience in the French military. Chapter 8 opens with an account of his return to civilian life, now in the Var town of La Ciotat. The final chapter considers Ramel by comparison with three other Midi physicians of the same era, Pierre-Joseph Amoreux (1741–1824), Esprit Claude François Calvet (1728–1810), and Michel Darluc (1717–83). The whole is summarized in the conclusions.

Biographies of famous French physicians and surgeons of the early-modern period are commonplace.[1] Written *consultations* and *consilia* by such individuals are also found in the archives.[2] Joël Coste contends that printed consultations were quite rare in the early-modern period.[3] Certainly, such works by lesser practitioners, and particularly those situated away from Paris, are rare, but Ramel did so, publishing in 1785 a series of medical consultations.[4] Gilles Barroux has described written consultations as, although not major, to be a significant form of medical exchange in the eighteenth century.[5]

Marie-François-Bernadin Ramel le fils was, and remains, one such less prominent individual in the context of French physicians of the late eighteenth century. I drew upon his consultations in *Medical Consulting by Letter in France, 1665–1789*.[6] In 2014, Joël Coste, in *Les Écrits de la soufrance: La Consultation médicale en France (1550–1825)* drew on Ramel's consultations, along with other French medical consultations, to analyse medical practices, patient sufferings, and the interaction between these.[7] Coste also included a very brief biography of Ramel.[8] Some of Ramel's publications were referred to in contemporaneous documents. In the *Encyclopédie methodique médicine par une société de médicins*, (1787) is a long article on Africa by M, Halle in which Ramel's publication on North Africa is extensively quoted.[9] Muriel Collart and Daniel Droixhe have examined Ramel's 1787 book *Aperçu et doutes sur la météorolgie appliquée à la médecine*, in the context of industrial pollution, pointing out that he was one of the first French physicians to question the connection between atmospheric conditions and disease.[10]

Brockliss and Jones have mentioned the casebook of physician Pellisier of St-Rémy-de-Provence [sic],[11] and Lisa Smith has written about the case books of Beaune physician Vivant-Augustin Ganiare (1698–1781); but these are exceptional as far as French country physicians are concerned.[12] The names of neither Pallisier nor Ganiare appear in the records of the *Académie royale de médicine* as contributing to the France-wide studies of the connection between weather and illnesses, a topic of significance to Ramel. Notwithstanding this, Ganiere was conscious of the impact of climate on his patients.[13] This was a field to which Ramel was drawn. Daniel Droixhe has considered the correspondence of a number of individual physicians, surgeons, and charlatans across France in the context of defining and treating cancer.[14]

Laurence Brockliss has investigated the life of Avignon physician Esprit Claude François Calvet and Montpellier physician-turned naturalist Pierre-Joseph Amoreux.[15] Brockliss has also made a brief comparison between Calvet and Amoreux.[16] Alain Collomp has written on the life of Michel Darluc, another rural physician-turned professor of natural history.[17] The similarities and differences between the lives of Ramel, Amoreux, Calvet, and Darluc are considered later. What light does the biography and writings of Ramel throw on French medicine and society in the eighteenth century?

One aspect of Ramel's work, which is given prominence, is his interest in the influence of weather on illness. The topic of medico-meteorology was extensively studied in the eighteenth century. Brockliss and Jones attribute the commencement of the interest in the effect of air on the body to Joseph Raulin (1708–84).[18] Raulin who received his doctorate in medicine at Bordeaux, published in 1752 *Des maladies occasionnées par les promptes et fréquentes variations de l'air....*[19] He wrote:

> I have always observed since I started to practise medicine, that one pays too little attention to the prompt and frequent variations of the air, and that one cannot look at enough as one of the principle causes of illness.[20]

His argument was essentially developed from Hippocratic theory. In *On Airs, Waters and Places*, Hippocrates had contended:

> Whoever wishes to investigate medicine properly should proceed thus: in the first place to consider the seasons of the year, and what effects each of them produces for they are not at all alike, but differ much from themselves in regard to their changes. Then the winds, the hot and the cold, especially such as are common to all countries, and then such as are peculiar to each locality. We must also consider the qualities of the waters, for as they differ from one another in taste and weight, so also do they differ much in their qualities.[21]

Thus, although the contribution of climate to human disease came to the fore in eighteenth-century Europe, it had ancient roots.

James Riley has also examined the literature around the relationship between the environment and ill-health.[22] His argument is that the eighteenth-century 'physician would put the environment under surveillance in order to detect its disease-conducive qualities, and to discover how to avoid them'.[23] Andrea Rusnock examined early-modern publications on the relationship between the weather and disease in England and France.[24] As far as France was concerned, she drew particular attention to the work of Jean Razoux, which is discussed in detail later.

Notes

1 Jean Astruc (1684–1766) in his memoires on the history of the Montpellier faculty of medicine gave details about significant doctors at Montpellier from 1080 to 1756. Jean Astruc, *Mémoires pour servir à l'histoire de la faculté de médecine de Montpellier*, Paris, Chez P.J. Cavelier, 1767.
2 For example, Paul Joseph Barthez (1734–1806), Pierre Chirac (1648–1742), Charles Louis Dumas (1765–1813), Jean Fernel (1506–58), Antoine Fizes (1689–1765), Etienne-François Geoffroy (1672–1731), Antoine Louis (1723–92), Henri-François Le Dran (1685–1770), Louis-Jean Le Thieullier (d. 1751).
3 Joël Coste, *Practical Medicine and Its Literary Genres in France in the Early Modern Period*, Paris, Université Paris Descartes, 2008, p. 4.
4 François-Bernadin Ramel, *Consultations médicales et mémoire sur l'air de Gemenos*, La Haye, Chez Les libraires associés, 1785.
5 Gilles Barroux, *Philosophie, maladie et médecine au XVIII siècle*, Paris, Honoré Champion, 2008, p. 65.
6 Robert Weston, *Medical Consulting by Letter in France, 1665–1789*, Farnham, Ashgate, 2013.
7 Joël Coste, *Les Écrits de la soufrance: La Consultation médicale en France (1550–1825)*, Ceyzérieu, Champ Vallon, 2014.
8 Coste, *Les Écrits de la soufrance*, pp. 255–6.
9 M. Hallé, 'Afrique' in Vicq d'Azyr (ed.) *Encyclopédie méthodique médicine par une société de médecins* 14 vols., Paris, chez Packoucke, vol. 1, 1787–1830, pp. 281–353. M. Halle was probably Jean-Noël Hallé (1754–1822).
10 Muriel Collart and Daniel Droixhe, 'From Anti-climatology to Pre-industrial pollution. Retz, Ramel and the Medical Topographies Before the French Revolution', *Ympäristöhistoria, The Finnish Journal of Environmental History,* vol. 6, no. 1, 2016, pp. 16–28.
11 Laurence Brockliss and Colin Jones, *The Medical World of Early Modern France*, Oxford, Clarendon Press, 1997, pp. 537–8.
12 Lisa Smith, 'Secrets of Place: The Medical Casebooks of Vivant-Augustin Ganiare', in Elaine Leong and Alisha Rankin (eds) *Secrets and Knowledge in Medicine and Science*, Aldershot, Ashgate, 2011.
13 Ibid.
14 Daniel Droixhe, *Les charlatans du cancer*, Paris, Hermann Èditions, 2018.
15 Laurence Brockliss. *Calvet's Web*, Oxford, Oxford University Press, 2002 and Laurence Brockliss, *From Provincial Savant to Parisian Naturalist*, Oxford, Voltaire Foundation, University of Oxford, 2017.
16 Laurence Brockliss, 'La République des Lettres et les médecins en France à la veille de la Révolution: le cas d'Esprit Calvet', *Gesnerus*, vol. 61, 2004, pp. 254–81.
17 Alain Collomp, *Un médecin des Lumières: Michel Darluc, naturaliste provençal*, Rennes, Presses universitaires de Rennes, 2011.
18 Brockliss and Jones, p. 463.
19 Joseph Raulin, *Des maladies occasionnées par les promptes et fréquentes variations de l'air …* , Paris, Chez Huart and Moreau, 1752.
20 Ibid., p. viii.

21 Hippocrates, *On Airs, Waters and Places*, trans. Francis Adams, http://
   classics.mit.edu//Hippocrates/airwatpl.html.
22 James C. Riley, *The Eighteenth-Century Campaign to Avoid Disease*,
   Basingstoke, Macmillan, 1987, pp. 45–8.
23 Ibid., p. xi.
24 Andrea A, Rusnock, *Quantifying Health and Population in Eighteenth-
   century England and France*, Cambridge, Cambridge University Press,
   2002, pp. 109–36.

Bibliography

Astruc, Jean, *Mémoires pour servir à l'histoire de la faculté de médecine de
   Montpellier*, Paris, chez P.J. Cavelier, 1767.
Barroux, Gilles, *Philosophie, maladie et médecine au XVIII siècle*, Paris,
   Honoré Champion, 2008.
Brockliss, Laurence W.B., *Calvet's Web: Enlightenment and the Republic of
   Letters in Eighteenth-Century France*, Oxford, Oxford University Press,
   2002.
Brockliss, Laurence W.B., *From Provincial Savant to Parisian Naturalist*,
   Oxford, Voltaire Foundation, University of Oxford, 2017.
Brockliss, Laurence W.B., 'La République des lettres et les médecins en
   France à la veille de la Révolution: le cas d'Esprit Calvet', *Gesnerus*,
   vol. 61, 2004, pp. 254–81.
Brockliss, Laurence and Colin Jones, *The Medical World of Early Modern
   France*, Oxford, Clarendon Press, 1997.
Collart, Muriel and Daniel Droixhe, 'From anti-climatology to pre-
   industrial pollution: Retz, Ramel and the medical topographies before
   the French Revolution', *Ympäristöhistoria, The Finnish Journal of Envi-
   ronmental History*, vol. 6, no. 1, 2016, pp. 16–28.
Collomp, Allain, *Un médecin des lumières: Michel Darluc, natural-
   iste provençal*, Rennes, Presses universitaires de Rennes, 2011.Coste,
   Joël, *Les Écrits de la soufrance: La Consultation médicale en France
   (1550–1825)*, Ceyzérieu, Champ Vallon, 2014.
Coste, Joël, *Practical Medicine and Its Literary Genres in France in the
   Early Modern Period*, Paris, Université Paris Descartes, 2008.
Droixhe, Daniel, *Les charlatans du cancer*, Paris, Hermann Èditions,
   2018.
Hallé, M., 'Afrique' in Vicq d'Azyr (ed.) *Encyclopédie méthodique médicine
   par une société de médecins* 14 vols., Paris, chez Panckoucke, 1787–1830,
   pp. 281–353.
Hippocrates, *On Airs, Waters and Places*, trans. Francis Adams, http://
   classics.mit.edu//Hippocrates/airwatpl.html, Accessed 29.11.2016.
Ramel, Marie-François-Bernadin, *Consultations médicales et mémoire sur
   l'air de Gemenos*, La Haye, Chez Les libraires associés, 1785.
Raulin, Joseph, *Des maladies occasionnées par les promptes et fréquentes
   variations de l'air...*, Paris, Chez Huart and Moreau, 1752.

Riley, James C., *The Eighteenth-Century Campaign to Avoid Disease*, Basingstoke, Macmillan, 1987.

Roulston, Chris, *Narrating Marriage in Eighteenth-Century England and France*, Farnham, Ashgate, 2010.

Rusnock, Andrea A., *Quantifying Health and Population in Eighteenth-century England and France*, Cambridge, Cambridge University Press, 2002.

Smith, Lisa, 'Secrets of place: The medical casebooks of Vivant-Augustin Ganiare', in Elaine Leong and Alisha Rankin (eds) *Secrets and Knowledge in Medicine and Science*, Aldershot, Ashgate, 2011.

Weston, Robert, *Medical Consulting by Letter in France, 1665–1789*, Farnham, Ashgate, 2013.

2   Early Life

Marie-François-Bernadin Ramel was born in 1752 in Aubagne, a country town some 16 km from Marseille and 35 km from Aix-en-Provence. There had been a settlement there since at least the Gallo-Roman period, known as *Pagus Lucreti*, and the town derived its name from its health springs – *Ad Bainea* – in the colony of Arles. At the beginning of the eighteenth century it had a population of around 7,000, but with the plague outbreak of 1720, causing a death toll of 2,114, and with further poor crops and famine, the town declined.[1] By 1790 it had recovered to contain some 7,100 people.[2] Aubagne's economy was essentially agriculture-based – olives, grain, wine, and some fruits and vegetables. Most of the wine was exported to Italy. There were also a limited number of tanneries and potteries operating close by.

Marie-François-Bernadin Ramel was the only child of François Ramel (b. 1724) who practised medicine in the town for 50 years; his paternal grandfather had also been a physician.[3] The Ramel family had lived in the region for a considerable time and can be traced back to at least the fourteenth century; his great-grandfather had been described as bourgeois or merchant and at the beginning of the eighteenth century had on a number of occasions been *"consul de la commune"*.[4] Nothing seems to have been recorded about Ramel's father's practice. However, it must have been reasonably successful to have been able to afford to send his son to university. Ramel's mother was Claire Barthélemy whose family had also been established in the area for a long period. It is reasonable to assume that Claire's family were of the same social strata as the Ramel family.

It seems most likely that Ramel le fils' early education commenced at Leotard's Institution in Aubagne, from whence he proceeded to the *Collége de l'Oratoire* (*Collège de Saint-Marthe*) at Marseille.[5] With a population of over 100,000, Marseille was too far from Aubagne for Ramel to travel to and from each day, so he would have become accustomed to living in a much larger place than his home town. According to Grimaud (1909–93), this educational pattern was commonly adopted for the children of the Aubagne bourgeoisie.[6] Weight is added to this educational progress, as René-Nicolas Dufriche Desgenettes (1762–1837) in the 1790s described Ramel as student of the Oratorians.[7] Desgenettes qualified as a physician at Montpellier and was a military physician attached to the *Armée d'Italie* in which Ramel served when the two men met and conversed, as is discussed later. The Oratorian movement was a Roman Catholic sect founded by Pierre de Bérulle in 1611 and approved by the Pope in 1613. It had a fine reputation for providing a good education.[8] However, unlike the Jesuits, the Oratorian schools taught in French.[9]

From Marseille Ramel proceeded to the University at Aix-en-Provence. Aix was a provincial centre with a population of around 28,000. Given the family background in medicine, it is hardly surprising that he should head there to study medicine. It is quite likely that this is where his father had studied medicine, which would have aided Ramel's acceptance into the medical school. A medical faculty at Aix was first established in 1409.[10] Physician Victorin Laval (1848–1930) stated that an Aix student was required to undergo a minimum of two years study before sitting for the baccalaureate, prior to commencing a doctorate in medicine.[11] Under the 1707 Edict of Marly, a student had to study medicine for at least three years after the baccalaureate to obtain his degree.[12] Thus, he would have been in Aix for around five years. What Ramel would have been taught is less clear. Under the 1707 Edict of Marly, the curriculum at French schools of medicine was extended from physiology, pathology, and therapeutics to include anatomy, botany, and galenical and chemical pharmacy.[13] Widening the scope of the curriculum was a part of the monarchy's attempt to improve the quality of medical training.[14] Whether this was all provided and to what standard in a small faculty such as Aix is an unknown. However, his publications show that he was well versed in classical and contemporary medical literature. In his various writings Ramel only once referred to his time at Aix. That instance was when he claimed that during his studies, he had taken part in eleven autopsies at the Aix cemetery of patients suspected of dying of pleurisy.[15] Evidently his education was not solely book-based as there was a specific place for anatomical dissections. The medical faculty at Aix had had a professor of anatomy since 1462, and students could follow clinical teaching at the Hospital Saint-Jacques.[16] It is likely, as Charles Coury wrote, that "Life as a student could have been financially difficult but also happy because of the release of youthful energy in a collective environment".[17] The literature is contradictory on the cost of obtaining a medical degree. Brockliss and Jones, for example, state that at Montpellier it never exceeded 300–400 livres.[18] On the other hand Willem Frijhoff says that in Paris the cost was 5,614 livres in the mid-eighteenth century;[19] Paul Delauney quotes a case in 1746 when a Paris degree cost one individual 8,000 livres.[20] Charles Coury says the cost of a French medical degree was 5,614 livres in 1754.[21]

As indicated previously, his Aix study would have been a minimum of five years. According to Louis Barthélemy (1810–90), chef-lieu de baronnie d'Aubagne, Ramel obtained a degree in medicine at Aix, 18 July 1775.[22] Ramel was to state that he had been working in civil hospitals in Aubagne and La Ciotat for 20 years, which supports a date of 1774 for the completion of his degree.[23] Assuming he did finish his studies in 1774, it suggests he commenced his studies at Aix at the age of 15 years, not an unusual age to commence university studies in eighteenth-century France. As is detailed later, in December 1774 Ramel went to North Africa, which appears to be conflict with Barthélemy's claim that he obtained his degree in July 1775. Typically in France, the awarding of doctoral degrees was accompanied by much ceremony, including a student giving his professors gifts.[24] Either Ramel skipped this process, which seems unlikely, or, perhaps, he made a return trip to Aix-en-Provence for the purpose of partaking in the formalities. The number of medical students at Aix-en-Provence was small; in the decade when Ramel graduated it averaged only 2.6 medical doctorates per annum.[25] By an Act of 2 April 1663 of the Parliament of Aix, doctors of medicine from the University of Aix could practice anywhere in Provence without submitting to examination by another university.[26] Such privileges were of course liable to contestation outside Aix. In theory the Edict of Marly made a qualified doctor of medicine from a French university liable to pay a fee of 500 livres to practise in a region other than where he qualified.[27]

Thus, at around 22 years of age, Ramel's formal education ended. His pre-university schooling would have provided a foundation in classical Latin and philosophy. If there were limitations in the teaching of medicine at Aix-en-Provence, Ramel's post-university writing on a variety of medical topics would suggest that that this was not the case. He would have seen himself as now prepared to take on a professional role as a doctor of medicine. His first endeavour was to take up a position in North Africa, an unusual opportunity for one fresh out of university.

Notes

1 M. le Compte de Villeneuve, *Statistique du département des Bouches-du-Rhone*, Marseille, vol. 3, 1826, p. 352.
2 César Couret, *Histoire d'Aubagne: Divisée en trois époques principales*, Aubagne, Michel Baubet, 1860, p. 82.
3 Louis Barthélemy, *Histoire d'Aubagne: Chef-lieu de baronnie depuis son origine jusq'en 1789*, 2 vols., Marseille, Lafitte reprints (Réimpresion de l'édition de Marseille, 1889), vol. 2, 1972, p. 324.
4 Barthélemy, vol. 2, p. 323.
5 Barthélemy discussed the schools in Aubagne at this time, but did not mention Leotard's Institution. Barthélemy, vol. 1, pp. 322–33.
6 Lucien Grimaud, *Histoires d'Aubagne*, Aubagne, Lartigot, 1973, p. 59. Cited in *Dictionaire de journalistes (1600–1789)* Édition électronique revue, corrigée et augmentée du Dictionnaire des journalistes (1600–1789), p. 242.
7 René-Nicolas Dufriche Desgenettes, *Souvenirs de la fin du XVIIIᵉ siècle et du commencement du XIXᵉ ou mémoires du R.D.G.* 2 vols., Paris, chez Firmin Didot Frères Libraires, vol. 2, 1836, p. 316. Desgenettes became one of the most senior people in the French military health system.
8 For a description of the education provided by the Oratorians see Auguste Brun, 'Un collège d'oratoriens au XVIIIe siècle', *Revue d'histoire de l'Église de France*, vol. 35, no. 126, 1949, pp. 207–19.
9 *L'Oratoire de France*, www.oratoire.org/lhistoire-de-loratoire, Accessed 11.3.2018.
10 C. D. O'Malley (ed.), *The History of Medical Education, UCLA Forum in Medical Science*, No. 12, Los Angeles, University of California Press, 1970, p. 125.
11 Victorin Laval, *Cartulaire de l'université d'Avignon (1303–1791)*, Avignon, Seguina frères, 1884, p. 286.
12 *Édit du Roi, portant règlement pour l'étude & l'exercice de la médecine*, Registré en Parlement le 18 mars, 1707, p. 7.
13 Ibid., p. 9. Laurence Brockliss has described the teaching of medicine in early modern France, but did not specifically discuss the medical faculty at Aix-en-Provence, L.W.B. Brockliss, *French Higher Education in the Seventeenth and Eighteenth Centuries: A Cultural History*, Oxford, Clarendon Press, 1987, pp. 391–440.
14 Laurence Brockliss and Colin Jones, *The Medical World of Early Modern France*, Oxford, Clarendon Press, 1997, p. 500.
15 François-Bernadin Ramel, *Consultations médicales et mémoire sur l'air de Gemenos*, La Haye, Chez Les libraires associés, 1785, p. 406.
16 Charles Coury, 'The teaching of medicine in France from the beginning of the seventeenth century', in Charles Donald O'Malley (ed.) *History of Medical Education' UCLA Forum in Medical Sciences*, No. 12, Berkeley, California University Press, 1970, pp. 136–7.
17 Ibid., p. 129.
18 Brockliss and Jones, p. 483.
19 Willem Frijhoff, 'Graduation and careers', in Hilde de Ridder-Symoens (ed.) *A History of the University in Europe, Universities in Early Modern*

Europe (1500–1800), 4 vols., Cambridge, Cambridge University Press, vol. 2, 1992–2011, p. 362.

20 Paul Delaunay, *La Vie médicale aux XVIe, XVIIe, et XVIIIe siècles*, Paris, Éditions Hippocrate, 1935, p. 37.

21 Coury, p. 130.

22 Barthélemy, vol. 2, p. 324. There is an anomaly over the date that Ramel completed his doctorate, since, as is shown later, Ramel stated that he travelled to La Calle as a physician in December 1774.

23 On this author's behalf, an archival search was conducted on Ramel by the Service historique de la défense centre historique des archives, Vincennes. Ramel's time in Aubagne and La Ciotat hospitals is mentioned in Ramel's letter of 8 Feb. 1794 to Ramel de Nogaret. *'Depuis 20 ans [occupée] dans les hôpitaux Civils d'Aubagne et de la Ciotat*. Ramel de Nogaret (1760–1829) was unrelated to M-F-B Ramel.

24 See Natalie Zemon Davis, *The Gift in Sixteenth Century France*, Wisconsin, University of Wisconsin Press, 2000, pp. 47–8, and 80–1.

25 Dominique Julia and Jacques Revel, 'Les Étudiants et leur études dans la France moderne' in eid (eds) *Les universités européennes du XVIe au XVIIe siècle: Histoire sociale des populations étudiantes, ii*, Paris, 1989, 459–86. cited by Brockliss and Jones, p. 517.

26 Laval, *Cartulaire de l'université d'Avignon*, p. 286.

27 *Édit du roi*, pp. 11–12.

Bibliography

Barthélemy, Louis, *Histoire d'Aubagne : Chef-lieu de baronnie depuis son origine jusq'en 1789*, 2 vols., Marseille, Lafitte reprints, 1972 (Réimpresion de l'édition de Marseille, 1889).

Brockliss, Laurence W.B., *French Higher Education in the Seventeenth and Eighteenth Centuries: A Cultural History*, Oxford, Clarendon Press, 1987.

Brockliss, Laurance and Colin Jones, *The Medical World of Early Modern France*, Oxford, Clarendon Press, 1997.

Brun, Auguste, 'Un collège d'oratoriens au XVIIIe siècle', *Revue d'histoire de l'Église de France*, vol. 35, no. 126, 1949, pp. 207–19.

Couret, César, *Histoire d'Aubagne: Divisée en trois époques principales*, Aubagne, Michel Baubet, 1860.

Coury, Charles, 'The teaching of medicine in France from the beginning of the seventeenth century', in Charles Donald O'Malley (ed.) *History of Medical Education', UCLA Forum in Medical Sciences*, no 12, Berkeley, California University Press, 1970, pp. 121–73.

Davis, Natalie Zemon, *The Gift In Sixteenth Century France*, Wisconsin, University of Wisconsin Press, 2000.

Delaunay, Paul, *La Vie médicale aux XVIe, XVIIe, et XVIIIe siècles*, Paris, Éditions Hippocrate, 1935.

Desgenettes, René-Nicolas Dufriche, *Souvenirs de la fin du XVIIIe siècle et du commencement du XIXe ou mémoires du R.D.G*, 2 vols., Paris, chez Firmin Didot Frères Libraires, 1836.

Édit du Roi, portant reglement pour l'étude & l'exercice de la médecine, Registré en Parlement le 18 mars, 1707.

Frijoff, Willem, 'Graduation and careers', in Hilde de Ridder-Symoens (ed.) *A History of the University in Europe, Universities in Early Modern Europe (1500–1800),* 4 vols., Cambridge, Cambridge University Press, vol. 2 (1986), 1992–2011, pp. 355–415.

Grimaud, Lucien, *Histoires d'Aubagne,* Aubagne, Lartigot, 1973.

Julia, Dominique and Jacques Revel, 'Les Étudiants et leur études dans la France moderne' in *Les universités européennes du XVIe au XVIIe siècle: Histoire sociale des populations étudiantes,* 2 vols., vol. ii, Paris, Éditions de l'École des Hautes Études en Sciences Sociales, 1989, pp. 459–86.

Laval, Victorin, *Cartulaire de l'université d'Avignon (1303–1791),* Avignon, Seguina frères, 1884.

O'Malley, C.D. (ed.), *The History of Medical Education, UCLA Forum in Medical Sci*ence, No 12, Los Angeles, University of California Press, 1970.

Ramel, Marie-François-Bernadin, *Consultations médicales et mémoire sur l'air de Gemenos,* La Haye, Chez Les libraires associés, 1785.

Service historique de la défense centre historique des archives, Vincennes: Gautier letter of 14 March 1794.

Gautier letter of 20 Nov. 1793.

Letter to Ramel de Nogaret, 8 Feb.1784.

Commission de Sante, Officier de Santé proforma for Ramel dated 15 July 1793.

Villeneuve, le Compte de, *Statistique du département des Bouches-du-Rhone,* Marseille, Ricard, vol. 3, 1826 [This multivolume work was published from an xvii to 1940].

3 Ramel in North Africa

His formal studies completed, Ramel sailed from Toulon to North Africa in December 1774 as a physician.[1] His destination was Bône (now Annaba) and principally, La Calle (now El Kala). La Calle was a semi-autonomous principality of the Ottoman Empire under the control of the Dey of Algeria.[2] La Calle had been a source of coral since the medieval period. In 1692 France obtained a concession granting exclusive rights to exploit the coral fishery off Bône, and in 1714 this was renewed.[3] Bône was under the jurisdiction of Le Caïd de Bône. The French concessions at Bône, La Calle, and Collo were controlled by the *Compagnie royale d'Afrique* for more than 60 years.[4] This organization was formed in 1599 and given letters patent the following year by King Henri IV. Its role initially was to protect the port of Marseille, but in the seventeenth century it was given monopoly of trade and commerce at these sites and was independent of the municipality.[5]

Bône was some 13–14 hours march west of La Calle.[6] Collo was even further west. Bône and Collo were exclusively native towns and never French colonies, and the *Compagnie royale d'Afrique*, which operated trading posts there, was restricted to renting a house for its employees.[7] The vessel which carried Ramel across the Mediterranean, a distance of some 400 nautical miles, also took six "principal officers" and around 30 men, some soldiers, some coral fishermen. It appears a further 25 men also travelled in the party.[8]

Why Ramel went to North Africa can only be conjectured. Perhaps in his early twenties he saw this as a great adventure. He was probably introduced to the idea of going to the Barbary Coast by his uncle Gabriel Ramel (b. ca 1728). Olivier Lopez refers to Ramel le fils as Gabriel Ramel's son, but he was clearly his nephew.[9] Gabriel first went to La Calle and Bône in 1749 aged 21–22 years, to work for the *Compagnie royale d'Afrique*. At that time Gabriel was described as "knowing absolutely nothing but who promised to become a great subject of the Company".[10] That confidence was justified, as by 1779 he had taken over the functions of Director General of the Company.[11] Further to his standing in the Aubagne community, Gabriel was mayor of Aubagne from January 1789 to March 1790.

In 1741 the Marseille-based *Compagnie royale d'Afrique* was granted a monopoly for the export of wheat and particularly coral from La Calle.[12] In practise, the Company was managed by the *Marseille Chambre de Commerce*.[13,14] The Chamber was formed in 1599 to help local businesses take a unified approach to government as they were confronted with a myriad of regulations covering imports and exports and the associated taxes.[15] *The Encyclopaedia of Islam* (1986–89) gives a description of the traditional method of fishing for coral at La Calle.[16] In addition to exports, imported goods manufactured in Europe were sold through a shop in La Calle.[17] In 1767 the total establishment at La Calle was limited by regulation to 147 individuals. By 1765, it had grown to 217, including 30 soldiers, which was considered too large by the Company.[18] The chamber's monopoly was subsequently supressed in 1791 like all other French monopolies.[19]

Ramel le fils' position at La Calle is not entirely clear. The extant records of the Company make no reference to him being appointed officially at La Calle.[20] Neither is there any record of his being paid a salary. In the seventeenth century, a report was prepared setting out costings for maintaining the concessions in North Africa.[21] This called for a physician to be paid 400 livres per annum, compared with 300 livres for a surgeon.[22]

Lopez describes Ramel as being *un chirurgien* – a surgeon.[23] This description has to be discounted; Ramel would not have qualified as a surgeon as becoming one was outside the scope of the universities.[24] The Company of Surgeons in Aix-en-Provence opened a school of surgery in 1767, with six professors.[25] Ramel would have been aware of this development, as he was studying medicine at the time.

Given the superior status of a physician over a surgeon, it is unlikely that Ramel would have considered himself anything less than a doctor of medicine.

During the time Ramel was in La Calle, the hospital there was under the charge of surgeon-major (*chirurgien-major*), M. Melan. *Chirurgien-major* was a military title but was also used at French overseas hospitals. As there were soldiers based at La Calle the *chirurgien-major* may have been military personnel although he was paid by the Company.[26] At the time, the hospital at La

Calle was serviced by three surgeons.[27] According to Paul Masson (1863–1938) the Company had ruled that La Calle was to be serviced by a surgeon-major as head of the hospital, and two chaplains.[28] Neither Masson nor Jean-Louis-Marie Poiret, in their histories of the concessions, mentions a physician spending time at La Calle.[29] However, Bernadin Ramel records that he was there over a six-year period and evidently practised as a physician during this time. The various papers he wrote, and particularly in his book *De L'Influence des marais et des étangs* (An X), made a number of reference to patients he saw at La Calle and the diseases from which they suffered.[30] These patients were mainly fishermen, coral divers, and other French individuals at the settlement. Under a 1744 regulation on the management of the North African concessions, surgeons were required to provide assistance and medications to the native population, albeit they had to pay for this.[31]

He quickly discovered that the climate in the region was not wholesome to new arrivals: "A few days after our arrival in these marshy areas, the strongest men, the most vigorous, in the flower of their age, felt innervated, were plagued by a heaviness, lassitude, cramps, serious diarrhoea".[32] This applied to the officers and soldiers.[33] It appears that there were also problems relating to drinking the water. Ramel noted that those individuals who drank water suffered pains in the stomach and serious diarrhoea and were constrained to drink wine; many officers who drank wine in moderation needed to dilute it with less water.[34]

Shortly before Ramel's arrival, La Calle surgeon Jauffroy, then the resident *chirurgien major*, wrote

> I find my health deteriorating more because of fatigue and the continual attention that it is necessary to give to the sick; of which the hospital never ceases to swarm, and of which the place is infected.... I beg you to provide in winter someone else with a better health than mine and more talent.[35]

Ramel made some references to the diseases of the native population, and how they treated themselves, although he made almost no reference to them being treated in the hospital.[36] He wrote specifically of:

> the unfortunate hordes of nomads who lead a patriarchal life under the tents which they bring to the edge of [the] lakes and in the low and humid places which offers them the most pasturage.

One sees the men of a seemingly bodily nature fat and muscular, but weak, slack, phlegmatic [in a humoural sense], pale, anaemic and incapable of doing the slightest work.[37]

In another document, however, Ramel describes the men, in general, as "tall and well proportioned, with well-made legs and muscular".[38] In this case he appears to be describing Arabs, and perhaps the earlier description refers to Berbers as both races co-existed in North Africa.

Curiously, he made no mention of what the animals were for which they sought pasture. Animal skins were exported by the indigent populace through La Calle. He did note that the locals, "*indigenes*", occasionally used a rough red wine as a febrifuge, that is, to counter fever.[39] In a 1794 paper he described two Moors being treated for drunkenness, having acknowledged that, as a rule, their religion forbade the drinking of alcoholic spirits.[40]

For intermittent fever he noted three alternative treatments employed by the indigenes: plunging into cold water, drinking eau de vie, and eating an excess of a Spanish red pepper.[41] He also commented that "Amulets and talisman were the means of healing in which the indigenous people had a great confidence and with which sometimes they had great success". This proved "how great is the influence of the moral on the physical".[42] He did briefly discuss some of the disorders that Arabic women suffered, *fleures blanches* which was very common, and irregular menstruation although he makes no mention of treating them.[43] He also noted that women in North Africa were more prone to maligne fevers than were men.[44]

Ramel also noted the differences in dress that the indigenous people adopted compared with that of the Europeans. In a discussion on the relevance of dress to health, he commented favourably on local practise relative to the climate, In particular he noted that the locals covered themselves as much in summer as in winter.[45] In a final note on the native population, he at one point referred to "*La Peste...cette maladie terrible*" affecting their villages, suggesting that they were subject to the plague which was endemic in North Africa.[46] Charles Féraud (1829–88) frequently refers to outbreaks of *la peste,* particularly in 1784–85. In one instance he claimed the gates to La Calle were closed to prevent the indigenes from entering into the town.[47]

Whatever his status was at the North-African concessions, Ramel went there equipped to observe the weather as he stated that that twice a day for six years the barometric pressure was recorded.[48] In addition to a barometer, he took with him a thermometer, a

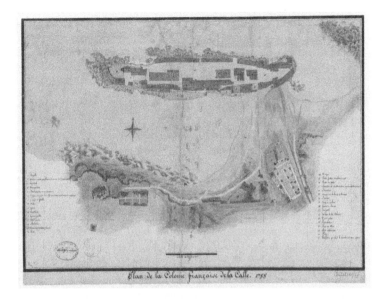

Figure 3.1 Eighteenth-century view of La Calle. Plan de la colonie française de La Calle, 1788. Courtesy: Bibliothèque nationale de France. Collection d'Anville; 08019 bis. https://catalogue.bnf.fr/ark:/12148/cb40592132k

eudiometer, and a hygrometer, although he did not state how often he took readings other than atmospheric pressure.[49] Nor did he indicate whether or not he took all the readings himself. Thus, it is evident that he proposed measuring atmospheric pressure, air temperature, the level of moisture in the air, and the ill-defined "goodness of the air". Apart from occasional references to temperatures, detailed records of Ramel's meteorological readings unavailable, but significantly in terms of the conclusions he drew, nor are details of exactly where he took measurements (Figure 3.1).

Geographically it is easy to envisage the North-African coast as largely sandy desert. Immediately around La Calle itself, this is the case, but moving a short distance inland, the area contained large lakes and swamps.[50] Ramel described the lakes thus:

> Three considerable lakes. The lake called Des Nadis which is to the east is divided into many small lakes and has no easily determined size. That of de St Jean the biggest and the nearest to La Calle, to the south, forms a very deep oval basin which is

about three leagues in circumference. The third which is to the western coast called Du Soug is divided into three or four small lakes of which the largest is about 120 steps in diameter, these lakes do not connect with the sea and mainly that of St Jean is the longest.[51]

La Calle is situated on coastal dunes but is surrounded by a heavily vegetated area comprising marshes, meadows, and forests. The lakes have a combined area of some 14,000 acres.[52]

French interest in the connection between meteorology and health took off in the 1750s and became what Brockliss and Jones have described as "initially a fad and ultimately an obsession".[53] Ramel evidently was initially infected by this enthusiasm.

Dario Camuffo and Chiara Bertollin have claimed the earliest systematic temperature observations were made in the period 1654–70 in two locations in Italy.[54] Muriel Collart has written on the history of the development of meteorology in the early-modern period. Whilst a number of these recordings were made by physicians, Collart's material makes no direct reference to the relationship between meteorological events and health.[55]

A prime example of the records that were compiled were those of Nîmes physician Jean Razoux (1723–98). Like his father, Razoux obtained his doctorate in medicine at Montpellier. As soon as he started working at the Nîmes hospital, L' hôtel-Dieu de Nîmes in June 1757, he commenced recording the temperature at the hospital twice daily as well as atmospheric pressure, wind direction and strength, the cloud conditions, and whether or not it had rained. The hospital had male and female wards for which he recorded daily the number of patients, how many were cured, how many died, and how many were in convalescence.[56] To complete the records he detailed the ailments from which the patients suffered, for the most part using the nosology of François de Boissier Sauvages (1706–67) and some information on treatment.[57] Razoux made monthly summaries of his data, the whole constituting a comprehensive record. In 1767, he published tables of his results, which covered most of the period June 1757–December 1761.[58] However, he did not attempt to make the direct connection between his medical data and the weather as many meteorological physicians did:

> By consulting these tables one can know what was the temperature of a season, and the dominant illness; if it was deadly, and until when; which are the most common illnesses in this climate,

if they are fatal or not; what is the danger to those who are attacked; which is the treatment that gave the most success ... One can also extract other advantages from these tables, on which I never insist, and that one can catch sight of at first glance.[59]

He wrote that when he commenced collecting this data it was not with the intention of it being published.[60]

Razoux's professional profile shows that he was much more than a rural doctor. He was a regular contributor to the *Journal de médecine, chirurgie, pharmacie etc*, over the years 1756–75. He was an associate of the *Société royale de médecine*, but unlike Ramel, he did not appear to have submitted entries when the society had offered prizes. Razoux was a member of the *Académie royale de Nîmes*, of which he was the perpetual secretary, and correspondent of the *Académie des sciences de Paris* and those of Montpellier and Toulouse.

Subsequent to Ramel's move to La Calle, such measurements took on a semi-official status. At the instigation of Anne Robert Jacques Turgot (1727–81), Controller General of Finances; the King's principal physician François De Lassone (1717–88); and anatomist Vicq d'Azyr (1748–94) in April 1776, order of the *Conseil d'État* required the setting up of a commission of medicine in Paris to establish a correspondence with rural physicians relative to climate and epidemics and epizootics.[61] The Society sought the clinical signs, diagnoses, and types of medications likely to stop such outbreaks, which country physicians encountered.[62] In 1778, the *Société royale de médecine* was formed with Vicq d'Azyr (1748–94) as its general secretary. Ramel took up the challenge to compile medical climatology and topography with zest. Large numbers of physicians, surgeons, and apothecaries across France collected and submitted records to the Society, which d'Azyr was to collate.[63] Jean-Pierre Peter counted some 150 medical practitioners who were correspondents, of whom about half "were faithful and regular".[64] The vast amount of data collected was never totally classified and analysed. This was the kind of project which appealed to Ramel. He reported to the Society on an epizootic at Aubagne in February 1784 and on an epidemic at Cassis in April 1790.[65]

This was just the sort of enterprise that seemed to appeal to Ramel. By travelling with a selection of meteorological equipment it is evident that he was of the view that it was worth studying the connection between climate and health. Ramel does not provide descriptions of his instruments, nor of where he obtained them. Vicq d'Azyr had reported in the 1790s that thermometers and barometers could not be bought in Paris or London.[66] In 1774 French meteorologist Père Louis Cotte (1740–1815) presented a treatise to the *Académie des science*, which included detailed descriptions of several varieties of meteorological instruments, including the types Ramel employed.[67] He also detailed precautions to be observed when these were used.[68] Muriel Collart has highlighted the difficulties encountered in the period when comparing data derived from differently constructed instruments.[69] As today, the results obtained in scientific measurements depend, amongst other things, on the apparatus employed. Ramel described Cotte as "the most celebrated meteorologist of our age".[70] To Cotte then, it was important when reporting results, to specify which instruments had been used to obtain meteorological data. In this regard, at least in terms of the available records, Ramel was imprecise.

It is almost certain that his thermometer was based on the Réaumur scale and was probably mercury filled.[71] Of the various thermometers and their associated scales which had been invented at the time, Réaumur's was French. Ramel identified his barometer as a mercury-filled instrument.[72] The hygrometer was most probably based on the length changes of a hair, but which fibre was involved is unknown. Ramel showed how up to date he was in science by also taking a eudiometer. This instrument was developed in the eighteenth century in various forms and was claimed to be able to measure the "goodness" or "healthiness" of air. Ramel gave no clues as to the construction of his eudiometer.[73] It was a contentious instrument, in part, because there was difficulty in obtaining reproducible results.[74] In 1785 the *Société royale de médecine* was reported as offering a prize of 300 pounds to the person who shall "ascertain the advantages which the practice of physic may be able to derive from the modern discoveries relative to the art of determining the purity of the air by different eudiometers".[75] The prize was awarded in August 1787, although I have not ascertained to whom, or the title of the winning dissertation.[76] A series of submissions by physicians was published as *mémoires* in the proceedings of the *Société*; the winner does not appear to have been Ramel.[77]

One instrument it appears Ramel did not take to La Calle was a rain-gauge, *pluviomètre*, yet when discussing intermittent fevers, he commented on the association between heavy rainfall and this type of disease.[78] Despite the large number of measurements he took, Ramel's records do not appear to have survived.[79] He made reference to his *Diarium practicum paludosum* in which he stated he recorded his daily observations in the hospital and the town in two quarto volumes. However, it is unclear which hospitals and towns he refers to, possibly those made in hospitals were in Aubagne and La Ciotat after his return to mainland France as well as at La Calle.[80] It does not appear that this document was ever published and the fate of these records is unknown; they have probably been lost. One would have hoped that compilation similar to that of Razoux had survived (Figures 3.2–3.5).

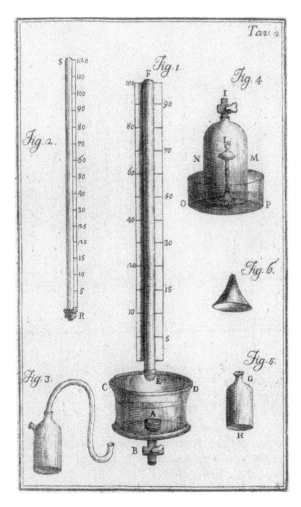

Figure 3.2 Example of an eighteenth-century eudiometer. Marsilio Ladriani, *Ricerche fisiche intorno alla salubrità dell'aria*. Milano: [G. Marelli], 1775. Courtesy: Wellcome Collection.

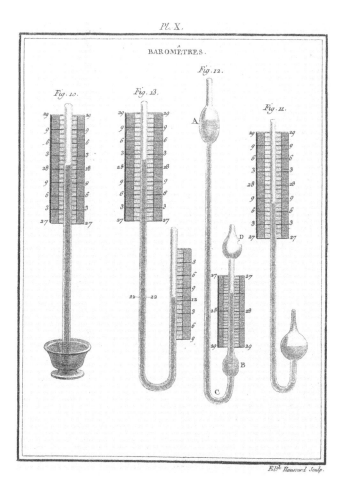

Figure 3.3 Some examples of eighteenth-century barometers. From Père Louis Cotte, *Traité de météorologie, contenant 1°. L'histoire des observations météorologiques...par le P. Cotte*, pl. 10. Courtesy: Bibliothèque national de France.

Over a period of time, Ramel had much to say on the topic of the relevance of meteorology on health and illness. In his 1785 book *Consulation choisies*, he remarked:

All ages of medicine had been marked by systems, less incorrect in themselves, than by the extension that is given to them. The system which characterizes the present age of medicine, is without

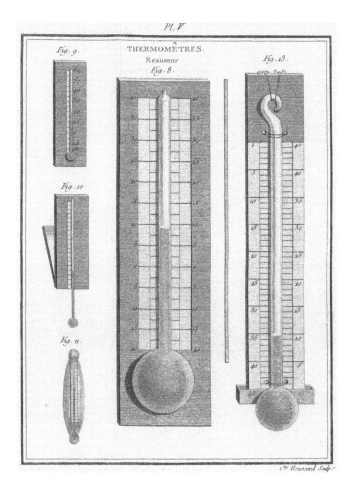

Figure 3.4 Some examples of eighteenth-century thermometers. From Père Louis Cotte, *Traité de météorologie, contenant 1°. L'histoire des observations météorologiques...par le P. Cotte*, pl. 5. Courtesy: Bibliothèque nationale de France.

doubt, the meteorological and constitutional system. The whole of the Republic of Medicine has its eyes fixed on the air. All the researches are aimed around these fluids. One attributes to them the generation of all illnesses. It has become the source [*artisan*] of all epidemics. Barometers, thermometers, hydrometers and eudiometers determine only some factors which would perhaps be more useful to our art, if they were directed towards other subjects.[81]

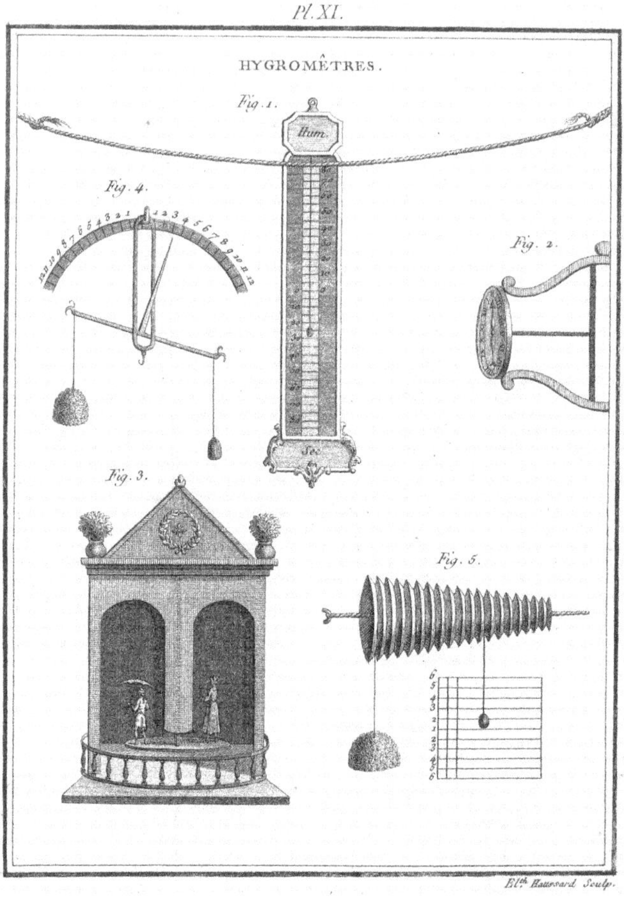

Figure 3.5 Some examples of eighteenth-century hygrometers. From Père Louis Cotte, *Traité de météorologie, contenant 1°. L'histoire des observations météorologiques...par le P. Cotte*, pl. 11. Courtesy: Bibliothèque Nationale de France.

In the same text he expounded in depth on the influence of air on the body under the heading *Memoire sur l'aire de Gemenos*. Gemenos is a small village some 5 km from Aubagne, with a population in 1793 of 1408. Set at the foot of a mountain it had different weather characteristics to Aubagne which lies in a valley, and Ramel was concerned with the consequential different health issues between the two locations. He opened this memoire with the claim:

Air has a singular ability to take charge of all the emanations of the body that it contacts and which it surrounds. These different emanations modify it and communicate to it [the body], good or bad qualities, relative to the dispositions in which one finds the animal that breathes it.

The very large extension that modern medicine has given to this principle, of which Hippocrates was the zealous advocate, itself started to have too great a generalisation, too distant to invalidate this doctrine, seems to the contrary to militate in its favour, and to prove at the same time that the human spirit easily proceeds further than the limits of truth.... This mass of pointless meteorological observations of which all the new works are replete, this amount of fastidious histories of epidemics about which the French press has complained for some years, without counting the epidemics of which many physicians prepare faithful histories for us, epidemics constantly and invariably attributed and related to the different atmospheric variations, without the alteration and the effect of the other six sorts of non-naturals are never blamed and seen as a predisposed cause, proving an irresistible extension that modern medicine gives to this principle.[82]

Ramel continued to discuss the properties of air and the factors which affected those properties, and, their effects on the human condition. He criticized contemporary doctors, "Physicians of today have made the air some common-place basket, or they choose for their arrangement the cause of all illnesses that they observe".[83]

Over time he had inconsistent views on the use of the hygrometer. In *De l'Influence des marais et des étangs sur la santé de l'homme* he advocated its value, claiming that he considered the hygrometer the most useful of instruments:

Of all the meteorological instruments, the hygrometer is without doubt the least known by physicians, and it is however the one which is the most necessary and most useful to them; we dare to say [it is] the only one which they must make use of because it is the only one capable of .... showing clearly the degree of humidity or of dryness of the local composition of the air where they exercise their profession, the make-up of which has the greatest influence on the life of the organism (*économie animale*).[84]

Whereas some four years earlier he had written in *Aperçu et doutes sur la météorolgie appliquée à la médecine*, that hygrometry was entirely useless in medicine.[85] Notwithstanding such inconsistences, it is clear that Ramel was familiar with current developments in medical science, and that he was of an experimental turn of mind. His work was not universally accepted. In a 1788 anonymous review of *Aperçu et doutes sur la météorologie appliquée à la médecine*, his conclusions were rejected:

> Thus, although the author of this dissertation discusses with much force and in depth the subjects which are material to it, his opinion on the absolute uselessness of meteorological observations, appear to us too positive & too divisive. It seems to us that he would have to modify it, & instead of advising abandoning this genre of observations, indicate a means of improving it.[86]

Ramel sought to be a part of the Republic of Letters, which meant that he had to expect his work to be open to criticism just as he criticized the work of others. One might regard this as the act of a man intent on upholding the ideals of the "Republic of Letters", even if it involved severely criticizing his own work. As this book was aimed at deriding the claims that meteorology could explain illness, it is possible that he was forestalling criticism that he had made the same argument. As noted previously he had stated that thermometric, barometric, hydrometric, and eudiometric observations were useless in medicine.[87] This book was also heavily criticized by Arras physician Noël Retz (1758–1810) who described Ramel's work as worthy of encouragement despite its many errors.[88] Despite this criticism, Retz had come to a similar position to Ramel's regarding the inadequacies of medical meteorology:

> A confusion of meteorological, topographical, nosological observations, and divisions of popular ailments, endemic, pandemic, sporadic, epidemic, intermittent etc.? But, what is the result of these multiple observations, often hazardous, disjointed and published with pomp, other than that amuses oneself, over 30 years, one has to draw from it some results even if of little significance, that we do not yet have one thing which is decisive & shielded from reproach or contradiction.[89]

Earlier in his career, Retz had been a proponent of such investigations.[90]

Ramel opened *Aperçu et doutes sur la météorolgie* with the comment that "The swamps and lakes exercise a tyrannical influence; oppressive and deadly to the health of men and animals".[91] This view was undoubtedly influenced, at least in part, by his North-African experience. In 1791 a paper of his was published in *Le Journal de médecine* on an epidemic of *angines* (pharyngitis) in La Ciotat.[92] Aside from describing the disorders, symptoms, and treatment, he compared the preceding and contemporary climatic conditions in La Ciotat with those at nearby Cassis, where there was no epidemic. He argued that there was no basis for attributing a meteorological cause to the outbreak. Indeed he lambasted the very notion:

> Yes, nature will always make light of such illusive pretentions and the puerile research of [medical] meteorologists, who work to trace a path that they cannot step aside from. It will always mock their vain efforts.[93]

Ramel was not satisfied with debunking false theories as a matter of opinion; he sought evidence to substantiate his arguments.

> Regardless that one brings to the examination of the phenomena that arise from air, and to their physical link relative to our bodies, some objection is the attention that one has to collect all that concerns this fluid [air], to examine many times a day the different variations of the barometer, the thermometer and the hygrometer, one will never come to the end of making meteorology, a certain and positive science, provide reliable rules on the action of air, and on its influence on the *économie animale*, to announce that some or other malady will follow some or other temperature or some or other atmospheric constitution.[94]

The arguments surrounding the relevance of meteorological medicine were to continue well into the nineteenth, even the twentieth centuries. For example, in 1853 *Association Medical Journal* published a series of articles, letters, and tables in which attempts were being made to associate atmospheric changes with the precise onset of disease.[95] In 2001 a group of physicians at the Wright-Patterson Air Force base in Ohio examined whether hospital admissions varied with climate changes, concluding that snowfall was the only significant factor of the parameters they analysed.[96] In October 2014

Deepak Bhattacharya presented a paper to the American Meteorological Society entitled "Medical Meteorology; Weather Assists Ease of Labour (Child birth) – a Unique Location in India" in which he argued that the effects of atmospheric pressure had a significant effect on labour.[97] But there are many others, showing the topic is still the subject of study.

It is evident that Ramel involved himself with the clinical aspects of the sick at La Calle as much as with his scientific measurements, after all, he sought to ascertain if there was a connection between local atmospherics and the diseases which were encountered. As previously noted, La Calle appears to have been an unhealthy place for French nationals. Fifteen percent of the letters between officers there and the Directors of the Company in Marseille between 1741 and 1793 relate to health problems.[98] He noted that men quickly fell ill on arrival at the settlement.[99] In a letter to the Company's directors of 3 November 1780, he claimed that there had been 33 deaths in the preceding ten months, although he did not detail the causes.[100] Ramel did publish some data on morbidity and mortality at La Calle, as shown in Table 3.1.

This data gives no idea of the nature of the illnesses involved in these summaries. Some further data specific to fevers is given later in his text.[101] How much time he devoted to treating the local populace is uncertain; however he made observations on their culture with respect to their illnesses. His time in North Africa, apart from practicing medicine, was occupied with examining the effects of the climate on disease. That he took instruments for this with him is evidence that he believed such investigations were worthwhile.

Table 3.1 Morbidity at La Calle for the years 1775–1781

Inside the hospital

Year	1775	1776	1777	1778	1779	1780	Total
Patients	1535	1451	820	1318	1595	1621	8340
Deaths	39	28	14	37	44	41	203
% Mortality	2.54	2.62	1.71	2.81	2.78	2.53	2.43

Outside the hospital

Year	1775	1776	1777	1778	1779	1780	Total
Patients	68	71	79	41	71	93	423
Deaths	3	9	12	18	15	16	73
% Mortality	4.41	12.68	15.19	43.90	21.13	17.20	17.25

Although, despite making many meteorological measurements, he appears to have become somewhat disillusioned with the use of some of the instrumentation he had employed. For whatever reason, the time had come for Ramel to leave North Africa and to establish himself in mainland France.[102]

Notes

1 Marie-François-Bernadin Ramel, *De L'Influence des marais et des étangs sur la santé de l'homme*, Marseille, Imprimeure-Libraire de J. Mossy, An X [1801/1802], p. 28.
2 Olivier Lopez, 'Les hommes de la Compagnie royale d'Afrique au XVIIIe siècle. Une intégration illusoire', *Cahiers de la méditerranée*, vol. 84, 2012, p. 53. http://cdlm.revues.org/6364, Accessed 02.07.2014.
3 Marxists Internet Archive: History Archive, Algeria, *Principal Dates and Time Line of Algeria 1501–1913*. www.marxists.org/history/algeria/1501-1913.htm. Accessed 19.01.2015 and Paul Masson, *Histoire des établissements et du commerce Français dans l'Afrique Barbaresque (1560–1793)*, Paris, Libraire Hachette, 1903, pp. 367–86.
4 Paul Masson, *Histoire des établissements et du commerce Français dans l'a Afrique Barbaresque (1560–1793)*, Paris, Libraire Hachette, 1903, p. 367.
5 For a detailed geography and history of the concessions see Laurent-Charles Féraud, *Histoire des villes de la province de Constantine. La Calle: et documents pour servir à l'histoire des anciennes concessions françaises d'Afrique / par Charles Féraud*, Algiers, V. Aillard et Cie, 1877.
6 Ramel stated the distance between La Calle and Bône was 15 leagues, but the league in France was not a fixed distance, so his 'march time' of 14–15 hours is probably more relevant.
7 Masson, p. 418.
8 Ramel, *De L'Influence des marais*, p. 28.
9 Lopez, fn., p. 52.
10 Masson, fn. 2, p. 428.
11 Lopez, p. 58.
12 Ibid., p. 49.
13 Masson, pp. 367–9.
14 For further details of commerce in the concessions see Le Baron Baude, *L'Algérie*, Paris, Arthus Bartrand Libraire, 3 vols., 1841, vol. 1.
15 Masson, pp. 367–71.
16 P. Bearman, Th. Bianquis, C.E. Bosworth, E. van Donzel, and W.P. Heinrichs (eds), *The Encyclopaedia of Islam*, 2nd ed, 12 vols., London, Brill, vol. 6, 1986–89, p. 556. 'Coral is said to be won [at La Calle] from a boat, a wooden cross, weighted with a stone, is sunk on a rope to the bottom of the sea; the boat sails up and down so that the corals get caught at the extremities of the cross, which then is weighed with a jerk. Then emerges a body with a brown crust, branched like a tree. On the markets these corals are abraded until they shine and show the desired red colour, then are sold in great quantities at a low price.'

17　Masson, p. 429.
18　Ibid., pp. 435–6.
19　Ibid., p. 548.
20　Archives de la chambre de commerce et d'industrie de Marseille-Provence. Hereafter referred to as A.C.C.I.M.P.
21　Sanson Napolon, *Estat de ce qui est nécessaire pour l'entretien du Bastion, La Calle, Cap de Rose, la Maison de Bône, d'Alger …* 'Cited by Charles Féraud, p. 135. This report was prepared by order of the King on the instruction of M. de la Villaubert, Secrètaire de ses Commandements en l'an 1626. Féraud, p. 129.
22　Baude, vol. 1, p. 386.
23　Lopez, p. 52.
24　One exception was at Montpellier where a joint degree in medicine and surgery was introduced, though rarely taken up. See Louis Dulieu, *La Chirurgie à Montpellier de ses origines au début du XIXe siècle*, Avignon, Les Presses Universelles, 1975, pp. 174–7.
25　Erwin H. Ackernecht, 'Some high points of the medical history of the Midi', *Canadian Bulletin of Medical History*, vol. 2, no. 1–2, 1985, p. 58.
26　Lopez, fn. p. 52.
27　Ibid., pp. 33–47.
28　Masson, pp. 429–30.
29　Jean-Louis-Marie Poiret, *Voyage en Barbarie, ou Lettres écrites de l'ancienne Numidie pendant les années 1785–6*, Paris, Chez J.B. F. Née de la Rochelle, 1789.
30　Ramel, *De L'Influence des marais*.
31　Féraud, Article 26, p. 326.
32　Ibid., p. 36.
33　Ibid., p. 38.
34　Ibid., pp. 38–9.
35　A.C.C.I.M.P. L111 392.
36　Ibid., pp. 131–3.
37　Ibid., p. 42.
38　Ramel, Bibliothèque Nationale de médecine, *Archives de la Société royale de médecine* Ramel, SRM 131B, no. 54, fol. 16. Hereafter references to these archives are listed as Ramel, SRM.
39　Ramel, *De L'Influence des marais*, p. 133.
40　Marie-François-Bernadin Ramel, 'Lettre du docteur Ramel au docteur Percy, chirurgien-major du dix-huitième régiment de cavalerie, associé de l'Académie de chirurgie de Paris, sur l'ivresse convulsive', *Journal de médecine, chirurgie, pharmacie etc.*, vol. 94, 1793, Paris, Didot le jeune, pp. 377–8.
41　Ramel, *De L'Influence des marais*, pp. 131–3.
42　Ibid., p. 130.
43　Ibid., p. 198 and 211.
44　Marie-François-Bernadin Ramel, *Aperçu et doutes sur la météorologie appliquée à la médecine*, Aix-en-Provence, Adibert, 1787, p. 168.
45　Ibid., pp. 284–5.
46　Ramel, SRM 131 B no. 54, fol.12.
47　Féraud, p. 310.

48 Ramel, *De L'Influence des marais*, p. 29.
49 Ibid., pp. 29–31.
50 See Edmond Lefranc, *La Calle, topographie, botanique et climatologie*, Paris, n.p., 1867, pp. 1–8. [Extrait du *Bulletin de la Société botanique de France*, 1862–65, vol. ix, pp. 423–30.] This also gives a description of the vegetation associated with the lakes which is seasonally variable.
51 Ramel, SRM131B, no. 54.
52 Lefranc, pp. 2–4.
53 Laurence Brockliss and Colin Jones, *The Medical World of Early Modern France*, Oxford, Clarendon Press, 1997, p. 463.
54 Dario Camuffo and Chiara Bertolin, 'The earliest temperature observations in the world: The Medici network (1654–1670)', *Climatic Change*, vol. 111, no. 2, 2012, pp. 335–63.
55 Muriel Collart, 'Prendre la mesure du temps : le réseau météorologique international de James Jurin (1723–35)' in in Pierre-Yves Beaurepaire (ed.) *La Communication en Europe de l'âge classique aux lumières*, 2014, Paris, Belin, pp. 76–86; and Muriel Collart, 'L'age d'or de la méteorologie dans la Mercure Suisse et le Journal Helvétique: le observations du doctuer Garcin', in Séverine Hugunin and Timothée Léchot (eds), *Lectures du Journal helvétique, 1732–1782, Actes du colloque de Neuchâtel*, 2014, Genève, Slatkine, pp. 269–91.
56 At the time Razoux was recording, Nîmes was a substantial city with a population of around 45,000, many times the size of Ramel's Aubagne. The city was home to a large garrison which resulted in a significant number of soldiers entering the hospital. James C. Riley, *The Eighteenth-century Campaign to Avoid Disease*, Basingstoke, Macmillan, 1987, p. 46.
57 François Boissier de Sauvages de Lacroix was a Montpellier physician and botanist who developed a system for the classification of diseases similar to that used by botanists based on symptoms and signs. See Louis Dulieu, 'François Boissier de Sauvages (1706–1767)', *Revue d'histoire des sciences et de leurs applications*, vol. 22, no. 24, 1969, pp. 303–22.
58 Jean Razoux, *Tables nosologiques & météorologiques tres éténdues dressées a l'hôtel-dieu de Nîmes*, Basle, Chés Jean Rodolphe Im-Hof et fils, 1767, pp. 80–256.
59 Ibid., pp. 12–13.
60 Andrea A. Rusnock, *Quantifying Health and Population in Eighteenth-century England and France*, Cambridge, Cambridge University Press, 2002, p. 129.
61 Jean Meyer,' L'Enquête de l'académie de médecine sur les épidémies', 1774–1794, *Études rurales*, no. 34, 1969, p. 7. In fact it was an outbreak of animal disease which prompted this move.
62 Ibid., p. 7.
63 Félix Vicq d'Azyr, *Mémoire instructif sur l'Etablissement fait par le Roi d'une Commission ou Société et Correspondance de Médecine*, Paris, 1776. *Les Archives de la Société royale de médecine* hold a large number of such reports from towns and cities across France. See Père Louis Cotte, *Résumé des observations météorologiques reçues par la SRM années 1777–1778, par le père Cotte*. SRM 194B dossier 29.

64 Cited by Harvey Mitchell, 'Rationality and Control in French Eighteenth-Century Medical Views of the Peasantry', *Comparative Studies in Society and History*, vol. 21, no. 1, 1979, pp. 83–4.
65 Ramel, SRM 180A, fols. 2 and 34.
66 Meyer, p. 13.
67 Cotte, pp. 99–210.
68 Ibid., pp. 521–8.
69 Collart, 'Prendre la mesure du temps'.
70 Ramel, *Aperçu et doutes sur la météorologie*, p. 72.
71 A number of scales were developed for measuring temperature. René Antoine Ferchault de Réaumur (1683–1757) invented his alcohol in glass thermometer around 1730; however, by the end of the eighteenth century, mercury had almost universally replaced the alcohol.
72 Ramel, *De L'influence des marais*, p. 29.
73 For a description of contemporary research on the use of the eudiometer see Marsilio Landriani, *Ricerche fisiche interno alla salubrita dell'aria*, Milan, n.p., 1775. Landriani provided diagrammes of the construction of his eudiometer as an appendix to this work.
74 For a description of the controversy surrounding the ability of the eudiometer to measure the goodness of air see Simon Schaffer, '*Measuring virtue*: Eudiometry, enlightenment and pneumatic medicine' in Andrew Cunningham and Roger French (eds) *The Medical Enlightenment of the Eighteenth Century*, Cambridge, Cambridge University Press, 1990, pp. 281–318.
75 The Society of Physicians in London, *The London Medical Journal*, vol. 5, issue 1, no. 3, 1784, p. 310. This English journal evidently converted livres into pounds.
76 M. Bru, *Méthode nouvelle de traiter les maladies vénériennes*, 2 vols. in 1, vol. 2, Paris, Chez l'Auteur, 1789, p. 286.
77 Pierre-Théophile Barrois (ed.), *Histoire de la Société Royale de Médecine: avec les Mémoires de Médecin : Année MDCCLXXXII et MDCLXXXIII*, 10 vols. Paris, chez Théophile Barrois le jeune, 1789, vol. 10, pp. 19–160.
78 Ramel, *De L'influence des marais*, pp. 93–4.
79 A.C.C.I.M.P. do not contain any such data.
80 Ramel, *De L'Influence des marais*, p. xvii.
81 Marie-François-Bernadin Ramel, *Consultations médicales et mémoire sur l'air de Gemenos*, La Haye, Chez Les libraires associés, 1785, p. 409.
82 Ibid., pp. 353–4.
    Ramel specifies six non-naturals other than air, yet traditionally there were only six including air, viz. air; motion and rest (exercise); sleeping and waking; food and drink; excretion and passions/ emotions.
83 Ramel, *Consultations*, p. 360.
84 Ramel, *De L'influence des marais,* p. 31. The term, *économie animale* unified physical and moral aspects of the study of man.
85 M.-F.-B. Ramel le fils, *Aperçu et doutes sur la météorologie*, p. 103. Ramel dedicated this work to his uncle Gabriel Ramel. Ibid., pp. 1–2.

86 *Journal de médecine, chirurgie, pharmacie etc.*, vol. LXXIV, janvier 1788, Paris, Croullebois, p. 174.
87 Ramel, *Aperçu et doutes sur la météorologie*, p. 103.
88 Noël Retz, *Nouvelles annales de médecine, chirurgie et pharmacie*, 5 vols., Paris, chez Méquignon, 1789, vol. 5, pp. 185–6. See also p. 39.
89 Retz, *Nouvelles annales de médicine*, vol. 2, pp. 15–16.
90 Nöel, Retz, *Météorologie appliquée à la médecine et à l'agriculture Par M. Retz*, Paris, Chez Méquignon, 1779.
91 Ramel, *De L'Influence des marais*, pp. 21–2. The book sold for 3 francs.
92 Marie-François-Benadin Ramel, 'Angines épidémique qui a régné â La Ciotat, durant l'hiver de 1791', *Journal de médecine, chirurgie, pharmacie etc*, vol. 88, August 1791, pp. 169–98.
93 Ramel, *Angines épidémique*, pp. 197–8.
94 Ramel, *Consultations*, p. 362.
95 *Association Medical Journal*, vol. 1, 1853, particularly no. 34, pp. 745–9.
96 Steven J. Durning, Lannie J. Cation, and Jonathon W. Buttram, 'Medical meteorology: Whether weather influences admissions', *Mayo Clinic Proceedings*, vol. 74, no. 4, 2001, p. 449.
97 Deepak Bhattacharya, 'Medical meteorology; weather assists ease of labour (child birth) – a unique location in India', *20th International Congress of Biometeorology*, Cleveland, OH, September 28–October 2, 2014.
98 A.C.C.I.M.P. Book 3, pp. 390–2, *Personnel des concessions*.
99 Ramel, *De L'Influence des marais*, pp. 36–7.
100 A.C.C.I.M.P. Book 3, pp. 390–2, *Personnel des concessions*.
101 See p. 53 below.
102 The French concessions in North Africa were largely closed in 1794 being privileged corporations. Féraud, p. 310.

Bibliography

Ackerknecht, Erwin H., 'Some high points of the medical history of provence', *Canadian Bulletin of Medical History*, vol. 2, no. 1–2, 1985, pp. 51–65.

Archives de la chambre de commerce et d'industrie de Marseille-Provence. Hereafter referred to as A.C.C.I.M.P.

Association Medical Journal, vol. 1, 1853, no. 34, pp. 745–49.

Baude, Le Baron Jean-Jacques, *L'Algérie*, 3 vols., Paris, Arthus Bartrand Libraire, 1841.

Bhattacharya, Deepak, 'Medical meteorology; weather assists ease of labour (child birth) – A unique location in India', *20th International Congress of Biometeorology*, Cleveland, OH, September 28–October 2, 2014.

Barrois, Pierre-Théophile (ed.), *Histoire de la Société Royale de Médecine: avec les Mémoires de Médecin: Année MDCCLXXXII et MDCLXXXIII*, Paris, chez Théopile Barrois le jeune, 10 vols., 1779–89.

Bearman, P., Th. Bianquis, C.E. Bosworth, E. van Donzel, and W.P. Heinrichs (eds), *The Encyclopaedia of Islam*, 2nd ed. 12 vols., London, Brill, 1986–89.

Brockliss, Laurance and Colin Jones, *The Medical World of Early Modern France*, Oxford, Clarendon Press, 1997.

Bru, M., *Méthode nouvelle de traiter les maladies vénériennes*, 2 vols. in 1, Paris, chez l'Auteur, 1789.

Camuffo, Dario and Chiara Bertolin, 'The earliest temperature observations in the world: The Medici network (1654–1670)', *Climatic Change*, vol. 111, no. 2, 2012, pp. 335–63.

Collart, Muriel, 'Prendre la mesure du temps: le réseau météorologique international de James Jurin (1723–35)' in Pierre-Yves Beaurepaire (ed.) *La Communication en Europe de l'âge classique aux lumières*, Paris, Belin, 2014, pp. 76–86.

Collart, Muriel, 'L'age d'or de la méteorologie dans la Mercure Suisse et le Journal Helvétique : les observations du doctuer Garcin', in Séverine Hugunin and Timothée Léchot (eds) *Lectures du Journal helvétique, 1732–1782, Actes du colloque de Neuchâtel*, Genève, Slatkine, 2014, pp. 269–91.

Cotte, Père Louis, Archives de la Société royale de médecine, *Résumé des observations météorologiques reçues par la SRM années 1777–1778, par le père Cotte*. SRM 194B, dossier 29.

d'Azyr, Félix Vicq, *Mémoire instructif sur l'Etablissement fait par le Roi d'une Commission ou Société et Correspondance de Médecine*, Paris, 1776.

Dulieu, Louis, 'François Boissier de Sauvages (1706–1767)', *Revue d'histoire des sciences et de leurs applications*, vol. 22, no. 24, 1969, pp. 303–22.

Dulieu, Louis, *La Chirurgie à Montpellier de ses origines au début du XIXe siècle*, Avignon, Les Presses Universelles, 1975.

Durning, Steven J., Lannie J. Cation, and Jonathon W. Buttram, 'Medical meteorology: Whether weather influences admissions', *Mayo Clinic Proceedings*, vol. 74, no. 4, 2001, p. 449.

Féraud, Charles, *L'Histoire des villes de la province de Constantin. La Calle: et documents pour servire à l'histoire des anciennes concessions français d'Afrique*, Algiers, V. Aillard et Cie, 1877.

Journal de médecine, chirurgie, pharmacie etc., vol. 94, 1793.

Journal de médecine, chirurgie, pharmacie etc., vol. LXXIV, January 1788.

Landriani, Marsilio, *Ricerche fisiche interno alla salubrita dell'aria*, Milan, n.p., 1775.

Le Franc, Edmond, *La Calle, topographie, botanique et climatologie*, Paris, n.p., 1867. [Extrait du *Bulletin de la Société botanique de France*, vol. ix, 1862–65, pp. 423–430].

Lopez, Olivier, 'Les hommes de la Compagnie royale d'Afrique au XVIIIe siècle. Une intégration illusoire', *Cahiers de la méditerranée*, vol. 84, 2012. http://cdlm.revues.org/6364

Marxists Internet Archive, *History Archive, Algeria, Principal Dates and Time Line of Algeria 1501–1913*. www.marxists.org/history/algeria/1501-1913.htm. Accessed 19.01.2015.

Masson, Paul, *Histoire des établissements et du commerce Français dans l'a Afrique Barbaresque (1560–1793)*, Paris, Libraire Hachette, 1903.

Meyer, Jean, 'L'Enquête de l'académie de médecine sur les épidémies', 1774–1794, *Études rurales*, no. 34, 1969, pp. 7–69.

Mitchell, Harvey, 'Rationality and control in French eighteenth-century medical views of the peasantry', *Comparative Studies in Society and History*, vol. 21, no. 1, 1979, pp. 82–112.

Poiret, Jean-Louis-Marie, *Voyage en Barbarie, ou Lettres écrites de l'ancienne Numidie pendant les années 1785–6*, Paris, Chez J.B. F. Née de la Rochelle, 1789.

Ramel, Bibliothéque de l'Académie nationale de médecine, *Archives de la Société royale de médecine (1778–1793)*, SRM Ramel, 180A, fols. 2 and 34.

Ramel, *Archives de la Société royale de médecine*, SRM Ramel, 131 B, no. 54, fols. 12, 16 and 54.

Ramel, Marie-François-Bernadin, *Consultations médicales et mémoire sur l'air de Gemenos*, La Haye, Chez Les libraires associés, 1785.

Ramel, Marie-François-Bernadin, *Aperçu et doutes sur la météorologie appliquée à la médecine*, Aix-en-Provence, Adibert, 1787.

Ramel, Marie-François-Bernadin, 'Angines épidémique qui a régné â La Ciotat, durant l'hiver de 1791', *Journal de médecine.chirurgie, pharmacie etc.*, vol. 88, August 1791, pp. 169–98.

Ramel, Marie-François-Bernadin, 'Lettre du docteur Ramel au docteur Percy, chirurgien-major du dix-huitième régiment de cavalerie, associé de l'Académie de chirurgie de Paris, sur l'ivresse convulsive', *Journal de médecine, chirurgie, pharmacie etc.*, vol. 94, 1793, pp. 366–88.

Ramel, Marie-François-Bernadin, *De L'Influence des marais et des étangs sur la santé de l'homme*, Marseille, Imprimeure-Libraire de J. Mossy, An X [1801/2].

Razoux, Jean, *Tables nosologiques et méteorologiques, très éntenduës dresées á l'Hôtel-Dieu de Nïmes*, Basle, ches Jean Rudolphe Im–Hoff & fils, 1767.

Retz, Nöel, *Nouvelles annales de médicine, chirurgie et pharmacy*, vol. 5, Paris, chez Méquignon, 1789, pp. 179–86.

Retz, Nöel, *Météorologie appliquée à la médecine et à l'agriculture Par M. Retz*, Paris, Chez Méquignon, 1779.

Riley, James C., *The Eighteenth-century Campaign to Avoid Disease*, Basingstoke, Macmillan, 1987.

Rusnock, Andrea A., *Quantifying Health and Population in Eighteenth-century England and France*, Cambridge, Cambridge University Press, 2002.

Sauvages de la Croix, François de Boissier, *Nosologie méthodique* 10 vols., Lyon, 1767, www.bium.univ-paris5.fr/histmed/medica/cote 31722X07. Accessed 09.01.2017.

Schaffer, Simon, '*Measuring virtue*: Eudiometry, enlightenment and pneumatic medicine', in Andrew Cunningham and Roger French (eds) *The Medical Enlightenment of the Eighteenth Century*, Cambridge, Cambridge University Press, 1990, pp. 281–318.

The Society of Physicians in London, *The London Medical Journal*, vol. 5, issue 1, no. 3, 1784, p. 310.

4   Return to Mainland France

Ramel recorded being at La Calle for six summers, meaning that he probably left permanently 1781, although he never indicated why he departed North Africa at that time.[1] One document refers to the number of patients in the La Calle hospital that year, implying that he was still there in 1781.[2] Whether or not he stayed in La Calle the whole time, or whether he made return journeys to mainland France during the six years, is never made clear, although the following case implies that he did make return trips. The earliest date encountered of a Ramel publication is 1778, concerning a young female with a displaced heart.[3] Somewhat curiously, although this was published as being by Dr Ramel fils at Aubagne, he was ostensibly in La Calle at this time. The woman was the daughter of a potter, and clay working was common in the Aubagne region. He also mentions the mother but not that he had discussed the case with her.[4] As French women were absolutely banned from going to La Calle, one has to presume he examined the patient in mainland France.[5] Masson has contended that the prohibition of women at La Calle was "because their presence could have been an occasion for troubles and insults on the part of the indigenous people".[6] The Abbé Poiret has described this regulation as a great cause of friction both to the men at the concessions and the women left on the mainland. He quotes one instance when a woman disguised herself as a man to get La Calle to join her husband.[7] In none of his publications does Ramel ever state that he treated indigenous women, although, as noted earlier, he was familiar with some of their medical complaints.

His years in North Africa would have given him experiences which he would have not found had he remained in Aubagne. As the only physician at the Concessions, at best he could only consult with surgeons if he wanted a second opinion on anything. Indeed, in his first year or so, he would probably have found it essential to draw on the experience of his surgical colleagues. It is likely that he would have had enough time to use his meteorological instruments and to ponder the relevance of the results he obtained, and how they related to disease. The apparent absence today of his records means that we have no way of knowing if he documented his conclusions whilst at La Calle; however, he had commenced corresponding with the *Société Royale de Médicine* by 1780, when he was ostensibly still at La Calle.

Ramel's permanent return to the mainland marked some significant events in his life. In France, parents had control over their children in matters of love and money. Chris Roulston has noted, "The age of majority ... in France [was] 25 years for women and 30 years for men".[8] So, it was on reaching this critical age that Ramel was emancipated by his father.[9] In 1782, he married Anne-Rose-Félicité Lieutard of Marseille.[10] Mme. Lieutard's father was a ship's captain, described by Ramel, "Parent, M. L. as a ship's captain who duelled with an Englishman. The Frenchman was victorious and the Englishman subsequently died. A few days later M. L. also died, of a malign fever, probably typhus".[11] Ramel does not give a date for this incident but says that it took place on a French American Island. In 1778, having recognized the United States of America as a sovereign nation, France signed a military alliance with the Americans and went to war with Britain.

With a wife to support, he needed to establish a source of income. This would not have been easy in Aubagne. With a population of around 7,000, it was already serviced by six physicians (including his father), and he would have made it seven, together with six surgeons, all competing to make a living.[12] It is almost certain that there would have also been an apothecary in the town.[13] This was an unusually high level of service, approximately one per 600 of the population, if one includes the surgeons. According to Sabine Barles, in France in 1786, there was on average one physician per 10,000 of population and one per 1,000 if one included surgeons.[14] Marc Rodwin has written that "in the 1770s French surgeons' fees were typically the daily wage of an agricultural worker or artisan, while physicians charged three times as much".[15] On the other hand, Brockliss and Jones state that "trained practitioners in small towns and villages must have been no better off than rich artisans, and in some cases in more parlous condition".[16] Places like Aubagne were too small to have a guild able to maintain either physicians' or surgeons' fees, as was often the case in larger towns. As will be noted later, Ramel le fils worked in hospitals in Aubagne and nearby La Ciotat, which presumably would have been remunerated.

This competetive scenario might be the reason for Ramel moving from Aubagne to La Ciotat, another small town (its population in 1793 was 6,160) some 16 km away, though precisely when is another uncertainty. A military record dated Brumaire An II (October 1794) states that he had been a resident of La Ciotat for eight years, which suggests his moving there in 1786.[17] In 1789 Ramel's contemporary Nöel Retz, in a critique of Ramel's book *Aperçu et doutes sur la météorolgie*, referred to Ramel as practising in La Ciotat.[18] Barthélemy says that he moved permananently to La Ciotat in 1789 or 1790.[19] In his various correpondences, Ramel often referred to himself as being *from* Aubagne, in the years 1783–92. It is of course possible that even when living and working in La Ciotat, he at times serviced patients in Aubagne. He recorded continuing his meteorological and clinical studies in the Western Var.[20] In medieval times La Ciotat was no more than a small fishing village. However, by the end of the eighteenth century a significant capability in building sailing ships had been established there with a consequent increase in population. His residency in the Var, be it Aubagne or La Ciotat, was interrupted by military service, of which more later.

The same year as he married, or perhaps 1783, the records are imprecise, Ramel undertook another overseas adventure. He recorded that he sailed to Minorca, a distance of around 270 nautical miles, on a captured vessel, at a time when France was at war.[21] Minorca had been ceded by Spain to the British under the 1712 Treaty of Utrecht. The Spanish, with support from the French, in part the Régiment de Bouillon, retook the island in 1782.This regiment moved on from Minorca to take part in the attempt by joint French and Spanish forces to also take Gibraltar. When this failed, the regiment withdrew to a garrison at Montpellier before moving to Besançon.[22] Ostensibly the reason for his trip was a quotidien fever which had persisted on the island for some months; however, Ramel noted,

> On arriving at Mahon, the fever had disappeared, without [the use of] any remedy. We experienced then that which many of the concesssionaires had related to us on the beneficial effects of a change of air. ... One knows however, ... that the air is not healthier, since [one] often sees prevailing there, illnesses analogous to those that one observes in the neighbourhood of swamps.[23]

In this context, it is reasonable to assume he is referring to those holding the North-African concesssions with which he was familiar. He did note, though, that there were many cases of intermitent fevers amongst English officers in the hospital of Mahon, the capital of Minorca.[24] One can only presume that Ramel returned from Minorca to the Var shortly afterwards. Nowhere does Ramel suggest that he had a formal role with the French army at this stage. His visit to Minorca is not mentioned in his military records so it is unclear what, or who, instigated this voyage.

Ramel noted that the regiment disembarked at La Ciotat prior to moving north and that on arrival at La Ciotat, a number of soldiers were suffering from *fievre maligne des prisons* – almost certainly typhus.[25] He pointed out that two physicians had died and that the disease took hold of the surgeons and nurses, and anybody who came close to the sick patients.[26] In one of his texts, Ramel noted that he had treated soldiers from this regiment at Aubagne as well as at La Ciotat, presumably because there was insufficient bed capacity at the latter.[27] La Ciotat had a history of dealing with sick soldiers. Historian Étienne Masse (1778–1862), who was born in La Ciotat, writing about the hospital there, stated that at least in the mid-eighteenth century it accomodated large numbers of soldiers in times of war. In the period February 1747 to February 1749 it handled 12,227 sick soldier days.[28] In 1788 Ramel commented that the La Ciotat hospital had 40 beds, and he considered it to be a model establishment.[29]

His return to mainland France saw significant changes in his life, getting married would have placed pressure on him to develop a regular income. Apart from whatever private practice he was able to undertake, which is indicated through his book of consulations, it is apparent that he worked in local hospitals. However, as is shown in the following chapter, Ramel also wanted to make a mark in the broader field of French medicine.

Notes

1 Marie-François-Bernadin Ramel, *De L'Influence des marais et des étangs sur la santé de l'homme*, Marseille, Imprimeure-Libraire de J. Mossy, An X [1801/2], p. 194, and again at pp. 144–5.
2 Marie-François-Bernadin Ramel Bibliothéque de l'Académie nationale de médecine, *Archives de la Société royale de médecine*, Ramel SRM 131B, fol. 33.
3 Marie-François-Bernadin Ramel, 'Observation de médecine, sur un cœur situé au – dessous diaphragme' par M. Ramel le fils, médecin à

Aubagne, prés Marseilles', *Journal de médicine, chirurgie, pharmacie, etc*, Paris, Ve Thiboust, no. 49, 1778, pp. 423–8.

4　Ibid., pp. 443–4.

5　Paul Masson, *Histoire des établissements et du commerce Français dans l'a Afrique Barbaresque (1560–1793)*, Paris, Libraire Hachette, 1903, pp. 443–4.

6　Ibid.

7　Jean-Louis-Marie Poiret, *Voyage en Barbarie, ou Lettres écrites de l'ancienne Numidie pendant les années 1785–6*, Paris, Chez J.B. F. Née de la Rochelle, 1789, p. 15.

8　Chris Roulston, *Narrating Marriage in Eighteenth-Century England and France*, Farnham, Ashgate, 2010, p. 9.

9　Prior to the Revolution, French parents exerted control over their children, including who could marry whom, was exerted up to the age to 30 years for males, and 25 for females, that is the ages of majority.

10　Louis Barthélemy, *Histoire d'Aubagne: Chef-lieu de baronnie depuis son origine jusq'en 1789*, 2 vols., Marseille, Lafitte reprints, 1972. (Réimpresion de l'édition de Marseille, 1889.), vol. 2, p. 324.

11　Ramel, *De L'Influence des marais*, p. 282.

12　Barthélemy, vol. 2, p. 321.

13　Barthélemy, vol. 1, p. 340, refers to the role of an apothecary servicing the poor who had to be a resident of Aubagne.

14　Sabine Barles, *La Ville Délétère : médecines et ingénieurs dans l'espace urbain XVIIIe–XIXe siècles, (Collection Milieux)*, Seyssel, Éditions Champ Vallon, 1999, p. 18.

15　Marc A. Rodwin, *Conflicts of Interest and the Future of Medicine: The United States, France, and Japan*, Published to Oxford Scholarship Online: May 2011, n.p. *Conflicts of Interest and the Future of Medicine: The United States, France, and Japan*, Oxford University Press, 2011; Suffolk University Law School Research Paper No. 11–16. SSRN: https://ssrn.com/abstract=1789751.

16　Laurence Brockliss Laurance and Colin Jones, *The Medical World of Early Modern France*, Oxford, Clarendon Press, 1997, p. 540.

17　Service historique de la défense centre historique des archives, Vincennes: Commission de Sante, Officier de Santé proforma for Ramel dated 15 July 1793.

18　Noël Retz, *Nouvelles annales de médicine, chirurgie et pharmacy*, Paris, chez Méquignon, 1789, vol. 5, p. 179.

19　Barthélemy, vol. 2, p. 326.

20　Ramel, *De L'Influence des marais*, p. 43.

21　Ibid., pp. 121–2.

22　*Histoire du Régiment de Bouillon*, http://users.skynet.be/michel.mordant/RegtBouillon.htm; users.skynet.be/michel.mordant/RegtBouil lon.htm.

23　Ramel, *De L'Influence des marais*, p. 122.

24　Ibid., pp. 121–2.

25　Marie-François-Bernadin Ramel, *Journal de médicine, chirurgie, pharmacie etc*, vol. 88, Paris, De l'Imprimerie de Monsieur, août 1791, p. 170.

26　Ibid.

27　Ramel, *De L'Influence des marais*, p. 170.

28 Étienne Michel Masse, *Mémoire historique et statistique sur le canton de la Ciotat: département des Bouches du Rhône*, Marseille, Caranud fils, 1842, pp. 217–20.
29 Bibliothéque de l'Académie nationale de médecine, *Archives de la Société royale de médecine (1778–1793)*, Ramel fils, SRM 175, *Topographie médicale de La Ciotat, Cereste, Cassis, Aubagne, Cuges, Gemenos, Roquevaire*, p. 15.

Bibliography

Barles, Sabine, *La Ville Délétère: médecines et ingénieurs dans l'espace urbain XVIIIe–XIXe siècles, (Collection Milieux)*, Seyssel, Éditions Champ Vallon, 1999.

Barthélemy, Louis, *Histoire d'Aubagne: Chef-lieu de baronnie depuis son origine jusq'en 1789*, 2 vols., Marseille, Lafitte reprints, 1972. (Réimpresion de l'édition de Marseille, 1889.).

Brockliss, Laurance and Colin Jones, *The Medical World of Early Modern France*, Oxford, Clarendon Press, 1997.

Histoire du Régiment de Bouillon, http://users.skynet.be/michel.mordant/RegtBouillon.htm; users.skynet.be/michel.mordant/RegtBouillon.htm. Accessed 29.11.2016.

Masse, Étienne Michelm, *Mémoire historique et statistique sur le canton de la Ciotat: département des Bouches du Rhône*, Marseille, Caranud fils, 1842.

Masson, Paul, *Histoire des établissements et du commerce Français dans l'a Afrique Barbaresque (1560–1793)*, Paris, Libraire Hachette, 1903.

Poiret, Jean-Louis-Marie, *Voyage en Barbarie, ou Lettres écrites de l'ancienne Numidie pendant les années 1785–6*, Paris, Chez J.B. F. Née de la Rochelle, 1789.

Ramel, *Archives de la Société royale de médecine*, SRM 131B, fol. 33.

Ramel, Bibliothéque de l'Académie nationale de médecine, *Archives de la Société royale de médecine (1778–1793)*, Ramel, SRM 175, *Topographie médicale de La Ciotat, Cereste, Cassis, Aubagne, Cuges, Gemenos, Roquevaire*.

Ramel, Marie-François-Bernadin, *De L'Influence des marais et des étangs sur la santé de l'homme*, Marseille, Imprimeure-Libraire de J. Mossy, An X [1801/2].

Ramel, Marie-François-Bernadin, *Journal de médicine, chirurgie, pharmacy etc.*, vol. 88, Paris, De l'Imprimerie de Monsieur, août 1791, p. 170.

Ramel, Marie-François-Bernadin, 'Observation de médecine, sur un cœur situé au – dessous diaphragme' par M. Ramel le fils, médecin à Aubagne, prés Marseilles', *Journal de médicine, chirurgie, pharmacie, etc.*, Paris, Ve Thiboust, no. 49, 1778, pp. 423–8.

Retz, Nöel, *Nouvelles annales de médecine, chirurgie et pharmacy*, vol. 5, Paris, chez Méquignon, 1789, pp. 179–86.

Rodwin, Marc A., *Conflicts of Interest and the Future of Medicine: The United States, France, and Japan*, Published to Oxford Scholarship Online: May 2011, n.p.

Rodwin, Marc A., *Conflicts of Interest and the Future of Medicine: The United States, France, and Japan*, Oxford University Press, 2011; Suffolk University Law School Research Paper No. 11–16. Available at SSRN: https://ssrn.com/abstract=1789751, Downloaded 08.02.2017.

Roulston, Chris, *Narrating Marriage in Eighteenth-Century England and France*, Farnham, Ashgate, 2010.

Service historique de la défense centre historique des archives, Vincennes: *Commission de Sante*, Officier de Santé proforma for Ramel dated 15 July 1793.

5 The Medical Savant

Ramel has already been shown to engage with the French medical establishment. The university-trained physician in the eighteenth century was an individual of some standing within society, particularly in small towns such as Aubagne and La Ciotat. It is clear that he sought to express his experience and knowledge beyond the small world of provincial Var towns. According to Lorraine Daston:

> [P]rior to the French Revolution concerns for personal glory greatly overshadowed concern for national glory among savants. Personal glory was more securely rooted in the essential nature of the Republic of Letters, in its worship of talent and its insistence on impartial judgement.[1]

The medical fraternity, despite community doubts about its ability to offer realistic cures and a sound theoretical basis for its practises, saw itself as being within the broad Republic of Letters. Ramel undoubtedly saw himself as a savant. Perhaps with time on his hands, and with an enquiring mind, he set about trying to establish a name for himself in the broader *"Republic de médecine"*, the term Ramel employed.[2] In 1785 he was elected a correspondent of the *Société royale de médicine*.[3] Furthermore, on numerous occasions Ramel noted that he was a corresponding member of the *Société royale de l'académie d'Arras*. He took to writing on matters medical. Ramel was unafraid to criticize fellow physicians when his evidence contradicted the theories of others even if they had established reputations. This was in keeping with the spirit of the enlightenment, that observed data and experiment should be disseminated, and if these contradicted prevailing wisdom, then so be it.

Ramel corresponded regularly with the Society, between 1783 and 1792 writing to it at least once a year on a variety of topics.[4] These letters and memoires post-date Ramel's return to mainland France from La Calle. As will be shown later, Ramel served for

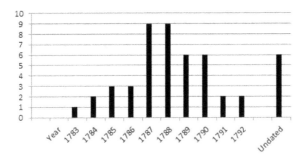

Figure 5.1 Frequency of letters from Ramel to the *Société royale de médicine.*[5]

three years in the French army, between 1793 and 1795. During which time he did not apparently correspond with the Society, nor afterwards (Figure 5.1).

He wrote not just about epidemics, but about the ailments of individuals, on plans to reorganize the provision of medical services in France, and even on the medical consequences of bread adulteration. In this last instance it was a complaint that certain bakers in Cassis were using *l'eau Saumatre* in their bread making a practice he considered fraudulent and dangerous. The term *eau Saumatre* was used for water, which was a combination of fresh and sea water and in consequence had a high salt content. As the bakers were already adding salt to the mix, the result was bread with, in his view, an excess of salt. Ramel contended that this was deleterious to a consumer's health.[6] Alongside Ramel's correspondence is a six-page response to the *Académie* from the mayoral office of Cassis, giving a detailed refutation of the claim that bread made in the town was unhealthy.[7] The correspondence ended some three months later in the form of a letter from Vicq d'Azyr, the Secretary of the *Académie*, which left the matter unresolved.[8]

Ramel wrote about the "Barbary scorpion" that he had witnessed at La Calle and Bône. He described it as so venomous that the victim of its sting could die within 24 hours. The victim suffered vomiting and convulsions, and when Ramel examined the corpse of a victim, he found black and purple marks where the bite had been but nothing else remarkable. He noted that this insect was common in all the towns and houses which were not well cleaned. His treatment was to apply "volatile alkalis", but he also recommended that theriac, in red wine, commonly regarded as an antidote for poisons, be taken internally.[9]

Ramel also involved himself with veterinary issues, when he wrote to the *Académie* about an outbreak of *morve* [glanders] amongst mules in Aubagne in 1783.[10] This infectious disease could be fatal in mules, affect other animals, notably horses, and even humans, so it was a matter of no small relevance. What most concerned Ramel was his inability to evoke any activity on the parts of the provincial veterinarian, or the bureau of police to whom he had to provide written reports on the outbreak.

On 11 March 1783, the Society proposed a prize of 600 livres, funded by the French King, on the subject:

> To specify which are the relationships which exist between the state of the liver and diseases of the skin; in which case the defects of bile, which accompany these diseases, which are the cause or the effect; to indicate at the same time the signs to be capable of knowing the influence of the signs one on the others, and the particular treatment that this influence demands.[11]

On 31 August of that year the Society announced that it was splitting the award, giving Ramel second prize, comprising a gold medal valued at 200 livres. The following month Ramel wrote to the society and thanked them, adding:

> The money and the sum that has been awarded to me will not be favoured by my grandchildren except that they had an ancestor who cultivated the sciences and who exercised with some distinction the most useful of arts. I prefer therefore the medal of 200 livres capable of allowing them to go back over the memory of my success and to inspire the love and virtue of the sciences. You will find attached the receipt of this medal.[12]

This was a desire of a man, at this time childless, but evidently expecting a continuation of his lineage. Ramel's letter suggests that his prize could have been 200 livres *or* a gold medal of equivalent value, and that he opted for the latter although this is not what the original documents indicate.

In 1784 Ramel published *Mémoire sur l'alipum, autrement di globularia*.[13] After a discussion on the uses of quinquina, a well-known febrifuge, he proposed the use of alipum as an alternative medicament. Whilst recognising the benefits of quinquina he was concerned that it was expensive and often adulterated and proposed Alipum as an alternative.[14] Alipum, which was native to the mediterannean region, was a febrifuge and mild purgative. As was common at the time for many natural medicaments, he claimed it could be of value in treating a wide range of conditions and as a tonic, giving details of which part of the plant to use, how it should be prepared and the appropriate dosages. On five occasions he prescribed it in his book of consultations described later. He claimed to have used it frequently with success in the Aubagne hospital, though noting it was ermployed differently in North Africa.[15]

The use of alipum was perhaps limited, as a major medical dictionary in 1817 noted that this plant was unknown to most physicians and one did not find it in other treatises on *materia medica*.[16] However, his article was cited not only in France but also in England as late as the second half of the nineteenth century.[17]

In 1784 he wrote a text based on some of his consulting cases, which was published the following year.[18] Forty-seven in all, a number of these cases were dealt with by correspondence, Ramel not having seen the patient. The practice of providing medical consultations by letter was commonplace throughout Europe, not least France in the eighteenth century.[19] Whilst a number of high-profile French physicians, and more rarely surgeons, published consultations in the eighteenth century, as a country physician, Ramel appears to be unique in this regard.[20] This book covered a range of disorders which he had encountered in his practice. He claimed that the principal purpose in publishing was to assist young, presumably meaning inexperienced, physicians. Whether the explanations he gave for publishing completely reflect his motivation is a matter for speculation. It is unlikely that he would have made much money from it.[21] It seems more likely, that he was trying to make a name for himself. It is also noteworthy that Desgenettes. Ramel's superior officer in the *Armée d'Italie*, describing Ramel's father as a wise and enlightened physician, who had contributed much to Ramel's publications.[22]

The diagnoses and therapies expressed in these cases were typically humoral, in line with the dominant medical theory of the period. The cases described were for the most part commonplace for the period, such as dysentery, melancholia, phthisis, and for women *"fleurs blanches"*, uterine haemorrhage, and chlorosis.

Less common ones included a case of *mal du pays*, a condition Ramel described as singular and rare.[23] Serious interest in this disorder followed the work of a French medical student studying in Basel, Johannes Hofer (1669–1752), who noted the frequent occurrence of it amongst Swiss mercenaries and coined the term nostalgia.[24]

Ramel described the suffering of persons from large cities, how they found the transfer to a country life debilitating after the lifestyle to which they were accustomed. What characterized this disease, how serious was it, and how could it be treated? Ramel detailed the condition of a 26-year-old patient. She had been happily married some six months, and her husband had taken her to the small town in which he lived. Her mother stayed with them some 15 days and then left for the family home. Some days later the young woman "... appeared less gay. Heavy clouds obscured the peacefulness of beautiful days ... she appeared reflective; eventually she became melancholic, she grieved about herself without reason, and lost her appetite. She suffered insomnia terribly". Her husband attributed it to her being pregnant; her local physician diagnosed *les vapeurs* and treated her accordingly, to no avail. Her brother went to see her for a few days, and she regained her gaiety and appetite, ceaselessly asking questions about her parents and other relatives in her home. When her brother left, she once more fell into sombre ideas and melancholy. Her brother consulted her doctor, who now diagnosed an *affection hysteriques* and prescribed accordingly. In his consultation, Ramel noted these remedies were of little use in such a case. He diagnosed her as suffering from *mal du pays*.[25] Along with the consultation Ramel published a letter from the patient's mother, who expressed her distress at her daughter's condition as well as the affection she felt for her daughter and son-in-law. In his reply to the mother, Ramel advised that often the treatments employed for *les vapeurs* would not work in this case of *mal du pay*. He assured her that her daughter could recover but that the mother "must disguise her affection to her daughter and neglect her to a point, so that she can do without you and rest with more pleasure beside her husband".[26] Ramel noted that to deal with such cases required understanding and to address the psychological causes.[27]

Another case he described concerned a man suffering from tetanus.[28] He wrote that this illness was more common in the North-African concessions than in Europe.[29] English physician Robert James (1703–56) described tetanus as most commonly caused by wounds and almost always fatal in the first three days.[30] After treatment by internal and external procedures, Ramel's patient was one of those fortunate to survive. His treatment did not include opium, despite his view in another work, *Aperçu et doutes sur la météorologie*, that "opium in very high doses was the only remedy for tetanus".[31]

As far as general therapies were concerned, Ramel employed the usual techniques of the period, although, he employed blood-letting less than some of his contemporaries.[32] Analysis of the therapies deployed in his published consultations shows the following (Table 5.1):

Table 5.1 Frequency of therapies prescribed in Ramel's published consultations

Therapy	Bleed	Purge	Enema	Laxative	Opiate	Emetic	Bathing	Waters	Lifestyle changes	Dietary restrictions
%	23.9	54.3	32.6	89.1	37.0	17.4	17.4	17.4	21.7	76.1

There were a number of unusual feature to this book. Firstly, he included the medical outcomes on the patients for whom he had provided advice.[33] Seldom did published French consultations tell the reader whether the proposed treatment regime had been successful or not.[34] Secondly, he used it as a vehicle to attack the work other physicians. It was not unusual for physicians to sometimes malign the efforts of surgeons, who they considered to be their inferiors, but not to openly criticize physicians.

It was almost universal for physicians and surgeons to condemn empirics and charlatans. On a number of occasions Ramel refers to the *"charlatan d'Arles"*. Although Ramel never named this individual, he was most probably the controversial Arles physician Pierre Pomme (1735–1812). The term charlatan was not normally applied to a qualified physician. Pomme had obtained his doctorate at Montpellier in 1747 and at one time was located in Paris as a court doctor.[35] Pomme's controversial standing arose from his publication *Traité des affections vaporeuses des eux sexes: ou Maladies nerveuses, vulgairement appelées maux des nerfs.*[36] Ramel railed against charlatans and empirics in general, as did every university trained physician.[37] But he was most vociferous about one local charlatan who he termed *"le Médecin aux pains cuits"*, because he prescribed a bread soup for every chronic ailment.[38] Such was Ramel's ire that he expounded a 251-word footnote detailing his criticism of this individual. Another he complained about for demanding payment in advance.[39] In 1789 he wrote to the *société royale de médecine* complaining of the activities of charlatans in small country towns.[40]

He made a vehement attack on the consultations of Louis-Jean Le Thieullier a well-regarded Paris physician who had died in 1751.[41] Ramel claimed that Le Thieullier's book "can only give some erroneous principles and a murderous practice to young physicians who will look to it for guidance".[42]

He also attacked a school of medicine, which issued degrees with little justification, except perhaps the fees charged:

It [Ramel's *Consultations*] will certainly be of more use for certain subordinate healers known in the Republic of Medicine, which are disowned, under the name of *Docteurs à la fleur d'O***. The odious corruption that [a] certain inexperienced university has allowed itself to licence medical qualifications, has given rise to a multitude of médicastres and empirics. As soon as that forgotten university, which assuredly merits its existence, opened its boutique to the ranks of assistant surgeons, who have only known to shave, and to crudely administer mercurial frictions, the assistant apothecaries who were only trained to give enemas and to mix some mercury, come running in a crowd to this market of qualifications... soon our region has been inundated by charlatans, empirics and médicastres.[43]

Medicastre was a pejorative term used at best for a bad physician, at worst a charlatan. Ramel was probably using the term *fleur d'O* rhetorically. It means a crown of orange flowers, and he is probably disparagingly comparing it with the doctoral bonnet. But further, as he goes on to attack an unnamed university. It is reasonable to suggest that this is a further play on words, intending to refer to the university at Orange. Laurence Brockliss and Colin Jones have described its medical faculty as "notoriously ... ready to award degrees after the most perfunctory examination".[44] Ramel almost certainly employed the term "boutique" satirically, perhaps even sarcastically. Despite his relative youth, Ramel was only 32 years old at the time, he was not reluctant to be outspoken. Joël Coste has regarded his criticisms of other practitioners, official or otherwise, as signifying Ramel's controversial character.[45]

Ramel was forward thinking in his approach to science, such as his attempt to get meaningful data from the use of a eudiometer. However he was not altogether taken by medical fads. He attacked, for example, the proponents of "animal magnetism" and the use of Mesmerism.[46] He accused the advocates of both, of claiming them to be panaceas, when in fact any patient response was purely mental. Indeed, Ramel was disparaging of all claims for universal panaceas. Thus, he disparaged the practise of an unnamed physician in the region of using the juice of chicory as a cure-all.[47]

One cannot help getting a sense from this book that Ramel had an underlying dissatisfaction with aspects of the way practitioners, in the broadest sense, and often his patients, attended to ill health. On the other hand as many of his epistolary consultations were in response to letters from surgeons, on a number of occasions he praised the way they presented information to him.[48] As noted previously he was prepared to criticize his own work; only two years after the publication of *Consultations*, Ramel remarkably wrote in his introduction to an article which questioned the value of meteorological medicine, that this work was useless.[49]

As noted previously he wrote about the atmosphere and its influence on the health of the inhabitants of Geminos. He contended that it was the air around the village that affected health, not the multitude of meteorological variables. Indeed, he remarked that the considerable increase in the population of Geminos over the period 1764–84 (the year he wrote the book) was proof of the healthiness of the air around the village.[50]

In 1785, it was Ramel's turn to criticize the work of Noël Retz in a letter to the *Société royale*. As noted earlier Retz had criticized some of Ramel's work; Retz had published a paper on the topic of diseases of the skin.[51] Whilst not directly accusing Retz of plagiarism, he hinted that this might have been the case.[52] He further suggested that Retz's claim to have invented a new type of hygrometer might also have been a copy of another physician's work.[53]

In 1787 Ramel published a second book, *Aperçu et doutes sur la météorologie appliquée à la médecine*. The main thrust of this book, whilst acknowledging the fundamental necessity of air to life, was primarily to criticize those who were bent on endeavouring to explain illness on the basis of meteorological data:

> At all points of the globe there are physicians and doctors who make their principal study the barometer, thermometer, hygrometer and eudiometer. If an epidemic occurs at one place or another, or another hemisphere, they never imagine that the bad quality or criminal falsifications of food, solid or liquid, that the passions, [and] finally the physical and moral habits of the inhabitants which have some affinity, some resemblance in their symptoms, some uniformity in their spread and some universality.[54]

For Ramel, the air was more important, in particular the "emanations" it contained, which were harmful and oppressive to man.[55] Ramel believed that the noxious fumes in the working environment of many artisans were the cause of illnesses. He listed tanners, leatherworkers, tallow founders, hatters, wig-makers, glass-makers, furriers, all blacksmiths and gave details of the particular diseases to which many of these workers were prone.[56] He used this point to again attack the use of the eudiometer, writing, "it is in these enclosed rooms that we again invite the meteorologists to come and place their eudiometers, in order admit to the uselessness of this instrument in medicine".[57]

In 1788 the *Société royale* proposed a prize on the topic of *Topographie médicale*. Ramel submitted a manuscript in August of that year entitled *Suite de la topographie médicinale re La Ciotat, Céreiste, Aubagne, Cuges, Gemenos, Roquavaire, et autres lieux par M. Ramel d'. en médecine*. for which, he was awarded third prize, the value of which was described as *"un jeton d'or"*.[58] Prizes in the form of jetons were regularly awarded by the *Société*. Today a number of such items exist in collections or are available on the market. They were not currency but clearly could have been sold for their high metal value.

In March 1789 *La Société royale* offered a prize on the subject:

> Determine by observation which are the diseases that result from emanations of stagnant waters and marshy land that may be for those who live in these environments, for those who work in their drying out, and what are the means of preventing them and of its to remedy it.[59]

Ramel was awarded a gold medal valued at 200 livre for his *mémoire* and although a copy of this does not appear in the *Société* archives, he subsequently published two years later as *Sur L'Influence des marais et des étangs sur le santé de l'homme* – "On the Influence of marches and lakes on the health of man"; this was to be his last published work. Not that everybody agreed with his conclusions: for example, in 1789 a comment made of this book was "This gentleman made many observations on the subject [the effects of marshy effluvia] on the subject in Africa, using various meteorological instruments with great judgement; but he attributes too much to the mere humidity of the atmosphere".[60] This critique gives rise to another conflict over dates; this article was published in London in 1789, whereas the book was ostensibly not published until 1801.

The *Académie nationale de médecine* holds two more manuscripts written by Ramel. The first is a *Mémoire Sur les maladies les plus communes a Bonne et La Calle comptoires principaux de La Compagnie Royale d'afrique par M. Ramel le fils D^{re} en Médecine*.[61] Unusually for Ramel, the document is undated; however, it contains references to 1778, 1779, 1780, and 1784, so one can presume that it dates at least from 1784. Furthermore it is not addressed to any individual, or the *Société royale de médecine*. It opens with a historical and geographical description of the Company's concessions. He describes La Calle as a small village, Bône, which he spells Bonne, as a small town, yet he gives no detail as to what structures and facilities existed at the latter. The bulk of this memoire is concerned with the common disorders which arose at La Calle, their symptoms and treatment, in particular, of intermittent fevers, putrid fevers, and more rarely malignant fevers. He noted that in the summers of 1778, 1779, and 1780, the most common endemic diseases were particularly numerous. He did not specify which these diseases were, but he undoubtedly was referring to the fever species he had already discussed. In each of these years there were 100 patients in the hospital, and around 40 deaths.[62] The cause of these illnesses he attributed to the fact that "lakes and marshes were emitting an unhealthy air, as it were, pestilential [and] charged with deadly miasmic particles which engendered the most unfortunate illnesses and particularly, the intermittent, putrid and malignant epidemic fevers".[63] The concept of "miasmic particles" as the source of many illnesses was a common theory at the time.[64]

It is worth mentioning that Ramel briefly mentions *"la peste"*, which he described as a terrible illness that recurs in the villages around La Calle. Varlik has written that "Plague was present in at least one location in the Islamic world virtually every year between 1500 and 1850".[65] However, Ramel makes no mention of plague cases in the concession hospital.

The second memoire is in two parts.[66] The first part is ostensibly a dissertation on *Solanum pseudocapsicum* L. or *Pomme d'amour vegitale*, a plant of the Solonaceae family. In fact, Ramel discusses the medicinal properties and gastronomic properties and uses of several of the Solonaceae, including belladonna, potatoes, tobacco, aubergines, and peppers.

The second part, [the two parts are written continuously] is also titled *Mémoire Sur les maladies les plus communes a Bonne et La Calle comptoires principaux de La Compagnie royale d'afrique*. This title is almost identical to that of the first document; indeed, the first two paragraphs of both are almost identical, word for word; however, the whole of this second part is much shorter than the former document.

In the *Mercure de France* of 5 March 1785 it was announced that Ramel had been awarded a prize of a gold medal by the *Société* during its seances August 1783 and August 1784 for a Mémoire *"Sur les maladies les plus communes à Bonne et à La Calle"*. It does not indicate the value of the prize.[67] In contradiction to these dates, it is recorded in *Mémoires de la Société royale de médecine* (1787) that the award was made on 15 February 1785.[68] Whether this refers to the first or second of these memoires is unknown. Perhaps the longer document was produced as an entry for the prize.

In 1791 he wrote to Vicq d'Azyr seeking clarification on a proposed treatise for which the *Société royale de médicine* was to award a first prize of 600 livres.[69] The proposal was concerned with the efficacy of treatments for mania amongst those who had not reached old age. Ramel viewed the terms employed in the proposal to be ambiguous. Whilst Ramel's letter is marked as being responded to, no copy of the reply appears to have survived. Significantly, the proposal does not seem to have progressed, probably due to the demise of the *société* in 1793.

Thus, Ramel made repeated efforts to establish himself as a savant in the Republic of Letters, or to use his preferred term, the Republic of Medicine. As a physician in a small country town in the south of France, he can be counted as being sucessful not only through the publication of his essays but also by the medals he was awarded.

His endeveours in the field of essay writing were to end abruptly when he became involved with the French army.

Notes

1 Lorraine Daston, 'The ideal and reality of the republic of letters in the enlightenment', *Science in Context*, vol. 4, no. 2, September 1991, p. 381. doi: 10.1017/S0269889700001010, Published online: 26 September 2008.
2 For example, Marie-François-Bernadin Ramel, *De L'Influence des marais et des étangs sur la santé de l'homme*, Marseille, Imprimeure-Libraire de J. Mossy, An X [1801/1802], p. viii.
3 Pierre-Théophile (ed.), Barrois, *Histoire de la Société Royale de Médecine: avec les Mémoires de Médecin: Année MDCCLXXXII et MDCLXXXIII*, Paris, chez Théopile Barrois le jeune, 10 vols., 1779–89, vol. 5, p. 23.
4 Bibliothéque de l'Académie nationale de médecine, *Archives de la Société royale de médecine (1778–1793)*, Ramel SRM 115B–204. A number of which were subsequently published in various issues of *Journal de médicine, chirurgie, pharmacie*. And, Ramel SRM 131B, no 54, fols 32 and 41.
5 Based on the archival holdings of the Académie nationale de médecine, Paris.
6 *Archives de la Société royale de médecine (1778–1793)*, Ramel SRM, 180A. fols 5–7.
7 Ibid., Ramel SRM 180A. fol. 8.
8 Ibid., Ramel, SRM 180A. fol. 9.
9 Ibid., Ramel, SRM 180A, fol. 4. Theriac was a polypharmaceutical that had been used for centuries for many ailments, but particularly poisoning.
10 Ibid., Ramel, SRM 180A, fol. 1.
11 La Société royale de médecine, *Histoire de la Société royale de médecine…, Avec les Mémoires de médecine et de physique médicale…*

tirés des registres de cette société Année 1784 et 1785, Paris, chez Théophile Barrois le jeune, 1788, pp. 3–4.

12 *Archives de la Société royale de médecine (1778–1793),* Ramel, SRM 180A, fol. 10.

13 François-Bernadin Ramel, 'Mémoire sur l'alipum, autrement de globularia', *Journal de médicine, chirurgie, pharmacie etc,* Paris, 1784, vol. 62, Didot le jeune, pp. 374–88.

14 Ibid., p. 378.

15 Ibid., p. 361.

16 Une société de médecins et de chirurgiens, *Dictionnaire des sciences médicales,* vol. 18 (GÉN - GOM), Paris, Panckoucke, 1817, p. 477.

17 See for example Carl Martius, 'On wild senna'. *Pharmaceutical Journal and Transactions,* vol. 16, 1856–57, p. 427.

18 Marie-François-Bernadin Ramel, *Consultations médicales et mémoire sur l'air de Gemenos,* La Haye, Chez Les libraires associés, 1785. In 1794 the population of Geminos was 1240, but Ramel states that it was much greater at the time he wrote his book (p. 390). The preface to this text is dated 1784, and publication was in 1785, however none of the consultations themselves are dated.

19 See Robert Weston, *Medical Consulting by Letter in France,* 1665–1789, Farnham, Ashgate, 2013.

20 Weston, p. 44.

21 See Lucien Febvre and Henri-Jean Maryin, *The Coming of the Book,* trans. David Gerard, Geoffrey Nowell-Smith, and David Woods (eds), London, NLB, 1976, pp. 159–66.

22 René-Nicolas Dufriche Desgenettes, *Souvenirs de la fin du XVIIIe siècle et du commencement du XIXe ou mémoires du R.D.G.* 2 vols., Paris, chez Firmin Didot Frères Libraires, 1836, p. 316.

23 Ramel, *Consultations,* pp. 25–34.

24 Jackie Rosenhek, 'Dying to go home', *Doctor's Review,* December 2008, n.p., Montreal, Parkhurst Publishing.

25 He quoted in Latin from Sauvage's *Pathology & nosology method* to support his conclusion. A French translation, François de Boissier Sauvages de la Croix *Nosologie méthodique,* 10 vols., Lyon, 1767. www.bium.univ-paris5.fr/histmed/medica/cote 31722X07, places this disorder under the heading *Bizarries.* vol. 7, pp. 237–41.

26 Ramel, *Consultations,* p. 34.

27 Ibid., p. 392.

28 Ibid., pp. 67–73.

29 Ibid., p. 393.

30 Robert James, *A Medical Dictionary,* 3 vols., London, J. Roberts, 1743–1745, vol. 3, n.p.

31 Ramel, *Aperçu et doutes sur la météorologie appliquée à la médecine,* Aix-en-Provence, Adibert, 1787, p. 110.

32 See Weston, pp. 163–7.

33 Ramel, *Consultations,* pp. 391–419.

34 Weston, pp. 196–200.

35 See Sabine Arnaud, 'Citation and distortion: Pierre Pomme, Voltaire and the crafting of a medical reputation', *Gesnerus,* vol. 66, no. 2, 2009, pp. 218–36.

36　This was initially published in 1760, and republished several times with significant changes.

37　Ramel, *Consultations*, p. 11.

38　Ibid., pp. 270–1.

39　Ibid.

40　Archives de la Société royale de médecine (1778–93), Ramel, lettre SRM 107, dossier 4 / pièce 187, *Depuis l'arrêt du 5 mai 1781, les charlatans se replient dans les petites villes dans les campagnes.*

41　Louis-Jean Le Thieullier, *Consultations de médecine*, 2 vols., Paris, Charles Osmont, 1739.

42　Ramel, *Consultations*, pp. xxv–xxx.

43　Ibid., pp. x–xi.

44　Laurence Brockliss and Colin Jones, *The Medical World of Early Modern France*, Oxford, Clarendon Press, 1997, p. 194.

45　Coste, *Les Écrits de la souffrance: La Consultation médicale en France (1550–1825)*, Ceyzérieu, Champ Vallon, 2014, p. 69.

46　Ramel, *Consultations*, pp. 323–4 and xxxii–vi.

47　Ibid., p. 101.

48　For example, Ramel, *Consultations*, pp. 95 and 261.

49　Ramel, *Aperçu et doutes sur la météorolgie*, p. 103.

50　Ibid., p. 390.

51　Noël Retz, *Des Maladies de la peau, de leur cause, de leurs symptomes, des traitements qu'elles exigent de ceux qui leur sont contraires*, Paris and Amsterdam, Méquignon l'aine, 1785.

52　Ramel's letter to the Society, Ramel fils, *Lettre avec en plus des Réflexions sur un ouvrage intitulé Traité des maladies de la peau par Retz, médecin du roi par quartier*, SRM 197 is undated and was subsequently published as M.F.B. Ramel, *Retz, Lettres de M. Ramel, médecin de Provence, a M. Retz, médecin de Paris*, Aix-en Provence, veuve d'Augustin Adibert, 1788.

53　For a history of early hygrometers see Dario Camuffo, Chiara Bertolin, Chiara Amore, Arianna Bergonzinni, and Claudio Cocheo, 'Early hygrometric observations in Padua, Italy, from 1794 to 1826, the Chiminello goose quill hygrometer versus the de Saussure hair hygrometer', *Climatic Change*, vol. 122, 2014, pp. 1–2.

54　Ramel, *Aperçu et doutes sur la météorologie*, pp. 9–10.

55　Ibid., p. 34.

56　Ibid., pp. 46–53.

57　Ibid., p. 54.

58　*Journal de médecine, chirurgie, pharmacie etc*, Paris, Croullebois, vol. 76, 1788, p. 528. The first and second prizes were gold medals each to the value of 100 *livres*. The *jeton* was a medal-like token with no face value, was not legal currency, and often was not inscribed.

59　*Journal de médecine, chirurgie, pharmacie etc*, Paris, Pierre-Théophile, vol. 9, 1790, p. ii.

60　*The Analytical Review or History of Literature, Domestic and Foreign*, n.p., London, January–April 1789, vol. 3, p. 500.

61　Archives de la Société royale de médecine (1778–93), Ramel, SRM 131B, no. 54.

62　Ibid., Ramel, SRM 131B, no 54, fol. 32.

63　Ibid., Ramel, SRM 131B, no 54, fol. 41.

64 See for example Brockliss and Jones, p. 726.
65 Nükhet Varlik, 'Plague in the Islamic World, 1500–1850', in Joseph P. Byrne (ed.) *Encyclopedia of Pestilance, Pandemics, and Plagues*, 2 vols. A–M, Westport, Greenwood Press, 2008, vol. 1, p. 519.
66 Ramel, SRM 131B, no. 53.
67 *Mercure de France*, Samedi 5 March 1785, p. 34. A search of the society records has not identified this prize.
68 *Mémoires de la Société royale de médecine*, Paris, Chez Theophile le jeune, 1787, p. 10.
69 Archives de la Société royale de médecine (1778–93), Ramel, SRM 131B, no 39. And *Histoire de la Société de médecine..., Avec les Mémoires de médecine et de physique médicale... Publié par l'Ecole de santé de Paris*, Paris, Didot le jeune, 1789, vol. 10, pp. viii–ix.

Bibliography

Arnaud, Sabine, 'Citation and distortion: Pierre Pomme, Voltaire and the crafting of a medical reputation', *Gesnerus*, vol. 66, no. 2, 2009, pp. 218–36.

Barrois, Pierre-Théophile (ed.), *Histoire de la Société Royale de Médecine: avec les Mémoires de Médecin: Année MDCCLXXXII et MDCLXXXIII*, 10 vols., Paris, chez Théopile Barrois le jeune, 1779–89.

Bibliothéque de l'Académie nationale de médecine, *Archives de la Société royale de médecine (1778–1793)*, Ramel, SRM 115B–204. A number of which were subsequently published in various issues of *Journal de médicine, chirurgie, pharmacie*. And, Ramel, SRM 131B, no 54, fol. 32 and fol. 41.

Brockliss, Laurance and Colin Jones, *The Medical World of Early Modern France*, Oxford, Clarendon Press, 1997.

Camuffo, Dario, Chiara Bertolin, Chiara Amore, Arianna Bergonzinni, and Claudio Cocheo, 'Early hygrometric observations in Padua, Italy, from 1794 to 1826, the Chiminello goose quill hygrometer versus the de Saussure hair hygrometer', *Climatic Change*, vol. 122, 2014, pp. 1–2.

Coste, Joël, *Les Écrits de la soufrance: La Consultation médicale en France (1550–1825)*, Ceyzérieu, Champ Vallon, 2014.

Daston, Lorraine, 'The ideal and reality of the republic of letters in the enlightenment', *Science in Context*, vol. 4, no. 2, September 1991. doi: 10.1017/S0269889700001010.

Desgenettes, René-Nicolas Dufriche, *Souvenirs de la fin du XVIIIe siècle et du commencement du XIXe ou mémoires du R.D.G.* 2 vols., Paris, chez Firmin Didot Frères Libraires, 1836.

Febvre, Lucien, and Henri-Jean Maryin, *The Coming of the Book,* trans.. David Gerard, Geoffrey Nowell-Smith, and David Woods (eds), London, NLB, 1976.

Histoire de la Société de médecine..., Avec les Mémoires de médecine et de physique médicale... Publié par l'Ecole de santé de Paris, 10 vols., Paris, Didot le jeune, vol. 10, 1789.

James, Robert, *A Medical Dictionary*, 3 vols., London, J. Roberts, 1743–45.

Journal de médecine, chirurgie, pharmacie etc., 98 vols., Paris, Croullebois, 1754–93, vol. LXXIX, January 1788.

Journal de médecine, chirurgie, pharmacie etc, vol. 9, Paris, Pierre-Théophile, 1790.

La Société royale de médecine, *Histoire de la Société royale de médecine…, Avec les Mémoires de médecine et de physique médicale…tirés des registres de cette société Année 1784 et 1785,* Paris, chez Théophile Barrois le jeune, 1788.

Le Thieullier, Louis-Jean, *Consultations de médecine*, 2 vols., Paris, Charles Osmont, 1739.

Martius, Carl, 'On Wild Senna', *Pharmaceutical Journal and Transactions*, vol. 16, 1856–57, pp. 426–7.

Mémoires de la Societé royale de médecine, Paris, chez Theophile Barrois le jeune, 1787.

Mercure de France, Samedi 5 March 1785.

Ramel, Marie-François-Bernadin, 'Mémoire sur l'alilum, autrement de globularia', *Journal de médecine, chirurgie, pharmacy etc.*, Paris, 1784, vol. 62, Didot le jeune, pp. 374–88.

Ramel, Marie-François-Bernadin, *Consultations médicales et mémoire sur l'air de Gemenos*, La Haye, Chez Les libraires associés, 1785.

Ramel, Marie-François-Bernadin, *Aperçu et doutes sur la météorologie appliquée à la médecine*, Aix-en-Provence, Adibert, 1787.

Ramel, Marie-François-Bernadin, Ramel fils, médecin à Aubagne (2 prix), *Lettre avec en plus des Réflexions sur un ouvrage intitulé Traité* as M.F.B.

Ramel, Retz, *Lettres de M. Ramel, médecin de Provence, a M. Retz, médecin de Paris*, Aix-en-Provence, veuve d'Augustin Adibert, 1788.

Ramel, Marie-François-Bernadin, *De L'Influence des marais et des étangs sur la santé de l'homme*, Marseille, Imprimeure-Libraire de J. Mossy, An X [1801/2].

Ramel, Bibliothéque de l'Académie nationale de médecine, *Archives de la Société royale de médecine (1778–1793)*, Ramel, lettre SRM 107, dossier 4 / pièce 187, *Depuis l'arrêt du 5 mai 1781, les charlatans se replient dans les petites villes dans les campagnes*.

Ramel, Archives de la Société royale de médecine: Ramel, SRM 180A, fols. 1, 4, 5–10.

Ramel, SRM 131B, no 54, fols. 32, 39, 41, 53, 54.

Retz, Nöel, *Des Maladies de la peau, de leur cause, de leurs symptomes, des traitements qu'elles exigent de ceux qui leur sont contraires*, Paris & Amsterdam, Méquignon l'aine, 1785.

Rosenhek, Jackie, 'Dying to go home', *Doctor's Review*, December 2008, n.p., Montreal, Parkhurst Publishing.

Sauvages de la Croix, François de Boissier, *Nosologie méthodique* 10 vols., Lyon, 1767 www.bium.univ-paris5.fr/histmed/medica/cote 31722X07. Accessed 09.01.2017.

The Analytical Review or History of Literature, Domestic and Foreign, vol. 3, London, January–April 1789, n.p.

Une société de médecins et de chirurgiens, *Dictionnaire des sciences médicales*, vol. 18 (GÉN - GOM), Paris, Panckoucke, 1817.

Varlik, Nükhet, 'Plague in the Islamic World, 1500–1850', in Joseph P. Byrne (ed.) *Encyclopedia of Pestilance, Pandemics, and Plagues*, 2 vols., Westport, Greenwood Press, 2008, p. 519.

Weston, Robert, *Medical Consulting by Letter in France, 1665–1789*, Farnham, Ashgate, 2013.

6   The Revolutionary Period

The medical profession took an active role in the revolution. Thomas Carlyle (1795–1851) wrote:

> Among the professions particularly active in the French Revolution, the lawyers and physicians are especially distinguished. Though they did not possess the same influence as the lawyers they nevertheless played a remarkable part in the stormy scenes of that stupendous creation of Europe.[1]

Dominique-Jean Larrey (1766–1842), who was to become the foremost military surgeon in France, is said to have led 1,500 medical students to the storming of the Bastille on 14 July 1789.[2] This number appears to be impossibly high, but the origin of Larrey's estimated headcount is unknown. Physicians, surgeons, and an apothecary were involved in the National Convention and its successor the Legislative Assembly in 1792.[3] Notable physicians who played a part in the revolution included Jean-Paul Marat (1743–93) and Joseph-Ignace Guillotin (1736–1813), best remembered for the introduction of the decapitating machine which bears his name. According to Carlyle, Marat was present at the storming of the Bastille:

> One poor troop of hussars has crept reconnoitring, cautiously along the quais as afar as the Pont Neuf: 'We are come to join you,' said the captain, for the crowd seems shoreless. A large-headed, dwarfish individual of smoke-bleared aspect shambles forward, opening his blue lips, for there is sense in him, and croaks: 'Alight, then, and give up your arms.' The hussar captain is too happy to be escorted to the barriers and dismissed on parole. Who was the squat individual? Men answer; it is Dr Marat, author of the excellent pacific *Avis au Peuple*.[4]

As well as being a physician and veterinarian, Marat took to publishing during this period. This included a newspaper put out under various names, but almost certainly this was what was referred to as *Avis au Peuple* above. Marat was a vociferous supporter of the revolting poor.

On the other hand, Colin Jones has contended of physicians that "The humdrum life of general practice seemed to insulate them from Revolutionary passions: it was as if clients came before commitment".[5] As will be shown, in this regard Ramel appears to be something of an exception as he adopted the ideals of the Revolution with zeal.

As elsewhere in Europe, early-modern medicine was at an official level, practiced by a hierarchy comprising, at the top physicians, below whom were surgeons and then apothecaries. The latter two were perceived as hands-on artisans trained through apprenticeships, compared with the university-trained physicians. All three, particularly in cities and large towns, were supported by corporations and guilds. At the same time there was a plethora of "unofficial" practitioners, ranging from mid-wives to charlatans. As the eighteenth century progressed differences in the areas of medicine which they operated became increasingly blurred and disputation between the groups became more intense even to court battles over claimed privileges and legal rights.[6]

Reform of the system was probably inevitable and became a foremost issue for the *Société Royale de Médecine* under the leadership of its secretary Vicq d'Azyr. Many members of the society made submissions to the *Société* dealing with the issue. A plan was drawn up which would have completely revised the medical profession including teaching and the unification of medicine and surgery at selected establishments. The society published its plan for the re-organization of French medicine in 1790,[7] and it was presented to the National Assembly 3 October 1791 by Dr Guillotin, who presided over the *Comité de salubrité* whose function included such matters.[8] However, such a grandiose scheme was not to eventuate immediately. The August 8 and September 15 decrees of 1793 by the National Convention completely overturned all medical organizations. Faculties, teaching organizations, faculties of medicine, colleges of surgeons and pharmacy, the Academy of Surgery, the Royal Society of Medicine; all of the scientific societies, all over France, were disbanded and closed.[9] Guilds were originally going to be abolished at the same time but in fact survived, if not in name, until March 1794.[10] The elimination of guilds would have had a more direct effect on surgeons and apothecaries than on physicians. An extract of the proposal dated 19 October 1791 was published in the *Journal de médecine, Chirurgie, Pharmacie*. It is presumably this draft proposal to which Ramel referred in his letter of 24 April 1791 to the *Société Royal*, in which he wrote that he had read the plan, but made almost no observations on its content and thrust.[11]

These changes could have had significant implications for Ramel's practice. On 17 March 1791 "the [National] Assembly decreed that anyone could be licensed to practice medicine or surgery upon the payment of a small fee".[12] The consequence of this was that ostensibly anyone could practice medicine even if they had no training at all. How this might have directly affected Ramel's practice is unknown, but it may have been influential in his decision to offer his services to the military where the role of physicians was clearly defined. On 1 July 1792, after the Assembly had acted to open the practice of medicine to all and sundry, Ramel wrote to d'Azyr, referring to the *Societé's* restructuring plan, yet made no criticism of what had actually taken place, largely praising the work that the *Société* had done in the past.[13]

The Revolution saw social turmoil across France and the Midi was no exception to this generalisation.[14] Michel Peronnet has contended that the southern temperament was the carrier of passion and violence, particularly if religion was involved.[15] Peronnet cited a number of comments made in the French newspaper, *Le Moniteur Universel*:

> It is wrong to accuse the Midi of being in a perpetual ferment. The hot heads of our southern provinces are more [than those of the north] susceptible to receive disastrous impressions ... The horrible scenes which do not cease to be renewed in our unhappy regions. It seems that an evil genie had wanted to take over the good nature of the men that inhabit these beautiful regions: the agitation is a need of their burning souls and the way is open to the deceitful, to the enthusiasts who want to abuse it. It was the cradle of the inquisition... the albigeos... sacrifices... there is a long history of crimes where the politic is enveloped in the mantle of religion.[16]

Riots broke out simultaneously across Provence in the spring of 1789.[17] Aubagne, like much of the region, was an extremely violent place during the revolutionary period; it was the location of a succession of lynching, murders, arson, and pillage.[18] According to Stephen Clay, there were 19 executions in Aubagne during the height of the Revolution.[19]

The Ramel family, as bourgeois, were potentially in a precarious position. For instance on 24 August 1792, an unruly civilian mob, ostensibly taking part in a farandole, burned down a number of properties including a country house of his uncle Gabriel Ramel.[20] Gabriel, now returned from La Calle, was mayor of Aubagne between January 1789 and March 1790, a position he lost when the municipalities in France were reorganized in the December of that year, as a result of a decree by the National Assembly.[21]

The Couret family were neighbours of the Ramels in Aubagne, who suffered at the hands of the revolutionaries. The head of the family was treated as an enemy of the Revolution, was imprisoned and was lucky not to be executed.[22] On 15 January 1794, revolutionaries who were rounding up "émigrés", came to the Couret house and were going to march off the mother and her four children. Heavily pregnant, Mme. Couret pleaded that she was unable to make a long march, probably to Marseille, and what would happen to her children? Successful in her pleas, she was allowed to stay in Aubagne and the eldest son, César, as a 12 year old, became responsible for his mother and his three siblings (soon to become four).[23] How the boy managed the situation much impressed Ramel, who as will be shown later, turned to César for his own son's education.[24] It is possible that Ramel did not directly witness these events, as he was serving with the *Armée d'Italie* in 1794, but became aware of them on his return to the area.

Despite it being his birthplace, Ramel was extremely critical of the Aubagnais writing in 1788:

> That it would be difficult to find in France a place which offers more vulgarity, more dissention, more hatred, more jealousy: I will say furthermore, more self-esteem, of haughtiness, opinionated without merit and without talent ....there are few towns in France as nasty as that of Aubagne... Its inhabitants live in the cafés, the smoking houses and the gambling schools.[25]

This contrasts with his description in the same manuscript of the men of nearby La Ciotat whom he described as honest and polite.[26] In contradiction to this, Charles Lourde (b. 1807) said that La Ciotat like Aubagne was in constant turbulence and agitation, with the town divided into two contesting camps.[27] M. Diedier, local historian of La Ciotat, quotes 9 March 1791 as the date on which troubles commenced in the town.[28] According to the Abbé Berthe, Ramel moved to La Ciotat in 1789, proved to be a supporter of the Revolution and was a member of the *Comité de surveillance from* 1794 until he joined the Italian military campaign.[29] Such committees were set up to monitor plots by suspected people and have them arrested. M. Diedier describes the formation of such a committee in La Ciotat at the beginning of 1794 in which Ramel was one of 11 members.[30] Donald Sutherland has outlined the activities of such a *comité* in Aubagne, which was probably similar to that in La Ciotat.[31] Earlier, in 1790, Ramel announced in a note the creation of a *Société de bienfaisance*, a philanthropic society.[32] Thirty individuals joined and subscribed 2,000 livres each; the beneficiaries were to be the poor. The proceeds were to be used to build two boats; he added that the municipal officers excited by this example joined together to build, at their own cost, a third boat. This is perhaps indicative of Ramel's concern for the underprivileged.

It was at about this time that Ramel became involved with the army, though whether as a direct consequence of the Aubagne conflicts is unknown. It could be that he felt personally threatened and decided to look for a safer environment. Alternatively, he could have been attracted by the opportunity to be more fully engaged in medecine, and finally, and perhaps most significantly, he was symapathetic to the revoloutionary ideals. La Ciotat historian Roger Klotz has remarked that Ramel adhered to the Revolution with a passion.[33] In a letter to the *Société royale de médicine* dated "15 germinal 1792 – l'an premiere de la Repub. Français" Ramel addressed Félix Vicq d'Azyr, the secretary, as *"citoyen et confrere"* and signed himself as *"citoyen et confrere"* as opposed to his previous conventional practise during the *ancien régime,* such as a letter again to Vicq d'Azyr, dated 1 June 1788, which opened as *"Monsieur et illustre confrere"* and closed with *"Votre humble et trés obessant serviteure".*[34] This may reflect his concurrence with revolutionary elimination of words with connotations of status, or it may simply be cautious political correctness.

Physician Alexis Pujol (1730–1804) noted that the *Société* had proposed a prize on 600 livres on the subject of pathologies and therapies for diseases of the skin. This was not awarded, but Pujol reported that Ramel had subsequently been awarded a medal for it worth 400 livres in 1786. Pujol commented that he had enjoyed an amicable correspondence and in 1790 had proposed they publish joint memoires, but that he had lost contact with him. Pujol feared that Ramel might not have survived the Revolution or had fled overseas.[35] As it happens he wrote this after Ramel had died.

In 1803 the regulation of medical practitioners was again amended, which formalized the difference between a physician (or surgeon) and a lower grade of practitioner, the *officier de santé*.[36,37] This was of significance to Ramel. The 1803 act limited the designation of doctor of medicine to those who had qualified in prescribed schools, which did not include Aix-en-Provence, where he had obtained his degree. Ramel was probably disappointed by the fact that when the University of Aix-en-Provence was reinstated in 1806, it did not include a faculty of medicine.[38] Although, according to Carol Summerfield, the school of medicine at Aix-en-Provence was allowed, by the government, to continue in the early nineteenth century.[39]

The French Revolution represented an outbreak of civil unrest on an unprecedented scale and exposed divisions within society. As a member of the "professional" class, one might have expected Ramel to be unsympathetic to the Revolution. On the contrary, as Couret commented, he was "wedded to the ideas of '89".[40] He retained that viewpoint until he died. It is reasonable to suppose that this idealism was a factor in his decision to offer his services to the military.

Notes

1 Thomas Carlyle, 'The physicians of the French revolution', *Journal of the American Medical Association*, vol. XXVIII, no. 11, 1897, pp. 514–15.
2 N. Panagiotis Skandalakis, Lainas Panagiotis, Zoras Odyseas, and John E. Skandalakis, 'To afford the wounded speedy assistance: Dominique Jean Larrey and Napoleon', *World Journal of Surgery*, vol. 30, 2006, p. 1393.
3 Wikipedia, *Liste des membres de la Convention nationale par département*. See also Colin Jones, 'The *Médecins du Roi* at the end of the *Ancien Régime* and in the French Revolution', in Vivian Nutton (ed.) *Medicine at the Courts of Europe 1500–1837*, London, Routledge, 1990, pp. 242–3.
4 Carlyle, p. 514.
5 Jones, p. 242.
6 For a detailed description of the reform process see Laurence Brockliss, 'Medical reform, the enlightenment and physician-power in late eighteenth-century France', *Clio Medica*, vol. 29, 1995, pp.64–112.

7 Société royale de médecine, *Nouveau plan de constitution pour la médecine en France présenté à l'Assemblée nationale par la Société royale de médecine*, Paris, 1790.
8 This committee had 29 members of whom 17 were of a medical background. It was set up by the National Assembly to broadly oversee the practice of medicine and public health.
9 In fact medical schools were re-instated in Paris, Montpellier and Strasbourg in December 1794 combining medicine and surgery.
10 Jonathan Simon, *Chemistry, Pharmacy and Revolution in France, 1777–1809*, Burlington, Ashgate, 2005, pp. 115–16.
11 *Journal de médicine, chirurgie, pharmacie etc.*, vol. 89, 1791, pp. 1–72.
   And Marie-François-Bernadin Ramel Bibliothéque de l'Académie nationale de médecine, *Archives de la Société royale de médecine (1778–1793)*, Ramel, SRM 180A, fol. 37.
12 David M. Vess, 'The collapse and revival of medical education in France: a consequence of revolution and war, 1789–1795', *History of Education Quarterly*, vol. 7, no. 1, Spring 1967, p. 73.
13 Ramel, SRM 180A, fol. 40.
14 'The term Midi used as a geogrphical, ethnological and anthropological location [was] of recent use at the time of the Revolution'. Michel Perronet, 'Naissance du Midi', in Jean Sentou (ed.) *Révolution et contre-révolution dans la France du midi 1789–1799*, Toulouse, Presses universitaires du Mirail, 1991, pp. 25–6.
15 Michel Peronnet, 'Le Naissance du Midi pendant le Revolution', *Historyka Studia metoloogiczne*, vol. 21, 1991, pp. 123–41.
16 Ibid., p. 127. Citing, *Le Moniteur Universel*, of 4 November 1789, 7 October 1790 and 12 November 1790.
17 Monique Cubells, 'Les Mouvements populaires du printemps 1789 en Provence', *Provence historique*, vol. 36, July–September 1986, pp. 309–23.
18 For a detailed description of the mayhem in revolutionary Aubagne See Donald Sutherland, *Murder in Aubagne: Lynching, Law, and Justice during the French Revolution*, Cambridge, Cambridge University Press, 2009.
19 Stephen Clay, 'Les réactions du midi: conflits, continuités et violences', *Annales historiques de la Révolution française*, vol. 345, no. 1, 2006, p. 73.
20 Louis Barthélemy, *Histoire d'Aubagne : Chef-lieu de baronnie depuis son origine jusq'en 1789*, 2 vols., Marseille, Lafitte reprints, 1972. (Réimpresion de l'édition de Marseille, 1889), vol. 2, p. 279.
21 César Couret, *Histoire d'Aubagne: Divisée en trois époques principales*, Aubagne, Michel Baubet, 1860, pp. 45–6.
22 Ibid., pp. 53–4.
23 Ibid., pp. 56–7.
24 Ibid., pp. 108–9.
25 Bibliothéque de l'Académie nationale de médecine, *Archives de la Société royale de médecine (1778–1793)*, Ramel SRM 175, *Topographie médicale*, p. 64.
26 Ibid., p. 23.
27 Charles Lourde, *Histoire de la révolution à Marseille et en Provence: depuis 1789*, 3 vols., Marseille, Chez Senés, 1838–39, vol. 2, p. 30.

28 Marius Deidier, *La Ciotat pendant la période révolutionnaire 1789–95*, La Ciotat, Impremerie du Vieux Moulin, 1961, p. 23.
29 Abbé L. Berthe, 'Les Assemblées provinciales et l'opinion publique en 1787–1788', *Revue du Nord*, vol. 46, no. 189, Avril-juin 1966, fn. p. 195.
30 Deidier, p. 23.
31 Donald Sutherland, 'Etude en Cas: le comité de surveillance d'Aubagne', *Rives nord-méditerranéenes*, http://rives.revues.org/574 ; DOI: 10.4000/rives.574, Accessed 18.10.2017.
32 Deidier, pp. 22–3.
33 Roger Klotz, L'Admiral Ganteaume et les Ciotadens', *Récherches régionales Côte d'Azure et contrées limotrophes*, vol. 5, 2010, n.p.
34 Ramel, *Archives de la Société royale de médecine (1778–1793)*, Ramel, SRM 180A, fols. 40 and 29 respectively.
35 Alexis Pujol, *Ouvres de médecine practique d'Alexis Pujol*, 2 vols., Paris, Chez J-B. Baillière et chez Béchet jeune, 1823, vol. 2, pp. 102–3.
36 Robert Heller, 'Officiers de Santé: the second-class doctors of nineteenth-century France', *Medical History*, vol. 22, no. 1, 1978, p. 27.
37 For a detailed description of the various steps taken to change the training and qualification of medical practitioners see Marie-José Imbault-Huart and P. Huard, 'Concepts et réalités de l'éducation et de la profession médico-chirurgicales pendant la Révolution', *Journal des savants*, vol. 2, no. 2, 1973, pp. 126–50.
38 Edwin H. Ackerknecht, 'Some high points of the medical history of provence', *Canadian Bulletin of Medical History*, vol. 2, no. 1–2, 1985, pp. 58–9.
39 Carol Summerfield and Mary Elizabeth Devine, *International Dictionary of University Histories*, Chicago, Fitzroy Dearborn Publishers, 1998, p. 418.
40 Couret, p. 108.

Bibliography

Ackerknecht, Erwin H., 'Some high points of the medical history of provence', *Canadian Bulletin of Medical History*, vol. 2, no. 1–2, 1985, pp. 51–65.

Barthélemy, Louis, *Histoire d'Aubagne: Chef-lieu de baronnie depuis son origine jusq'en 1789*, 2 vols., Marseille, Lafitte reprints, 1972. (Réimpresion de l'édition de Marseille, 1889.).

Berthe, L., Abbé, 'Les Assemblées provinciales et l'opinion publique en 1787–1788', *Revue du Nord*, vol. 46, no. 189, Avril-juin 1966, pp. 185–200.

Brockliss. Laurence, W.B., 'Medical reform, the enlightenment and physician-power in late eighteenth-century France', *Clio Medica*, vol. 29, 1995, pp. 64–112.

Carlyle, Thomas, 'The physicians of the French revolution', *Journal American Medical Association*, vol. XXVIII, no 11, 1897, pp. 514–15.

Clay, Stephen, 'Les réactions du midi: conflits, continuités et violences', *Annales historiques de la Révolution française*, vol. 345, no. 1, 2006, pp. 55–9.

Cubells, Monique, 'Les Mouvements populaires du printemps 1789 en Provence', *Provence historique*, vol. 36, July–September 1986, pp. 309–23.

Couret, César, *Histoire d'Aubagne: Divisée en trois époques principales*, Aubagne, Michel Baubet, 1860.

Deidier, Marius., *La Ciotat pendant la période révolutionnaire 1789–95*, La Ciotat, Imprimerie du Vieux Moulin, 1961.

Heller, Robert, 'Officiers de Santé: The second-class doctors of nineteenth-century France', *Medical History*, vol. 22, no. 1, 1978, pp. 25–43.

Imbault-Huart, Marie-José, P.Huard, 'Concepts et réalités de l'éducation et de la profession médico-chirurgicales pendant la Révolution', *Journal des savants*, vol. 2, no. 2, 1973, pp. 126–50.

Jones, Colin, 'The *Médecins du Roi* at the End of the *Ancien Régime* and in the French Revolution', in Vivian Nutton (ed.) *Medicine at the Courts of Europe 1500–1837*, London, Routledge, 1990, pp. 209–61.

Journal de médicine, chirurgie, pharmacie etc., vol. 89, 1791, pp. 1–72.

Klotz, Roger, 'L'Admiral Ganteaume et les Ciotadens', *Récherches régionales Côte d'Azure et contrées limotrophes*, vol. 5, 2010, n.p.

Lourde, Charles, *Histoire de la révolution à Marseille et en Provence: depuis 1789*, 3 vols., Marseille, chez Senés, 1838–39.

Perronet, Michel, 'Le Naissance du Midi pendant le Revolution', *Historyka Studia metoloogiczne*, vol. 21, 1991, pp. 123–41.

Perronet, Michel, 'Naissance du Midi', in Jean Sentou (ed.) *Révolution et contre-révolution dans la France du midi 1789–1799*, Toulouse, Presses universitaires du Mirail, 1991.

Pujol, Alexis, *Ouvres de médecine practique d'Alexis Pujol*, 2 vols., Paris, Chez J-B. Baillière et chez Béchet jeune, 1823.

Ramel, Marie-François-Bernadin, *Archives de la Société royale de médecine (1778–1793)*, SRM Ramel.180A, fols. 37, 40 and 29 respectively.

Ramel, Marie-François-Bernadin, Bibliothéque de l'Académie nationale de médecine, *Archives de la Société royale de médecine (1778–1793)*, Ramel SRM 175, *Topographie médicale*.

Simon, Jonathan, *Chemistry, Pharmacy and Revolution in France, 1777–1809*, Burlington, Ashgate, 2005.

Skandalakis, N. Panagiotis, Lainas Panagiotis, Zoras Odyseas, and John E. Skandalakis, 'To afford the wounded speedy assistance: Dominique Jean Larrey and Napoleon', *World Journal of Surgery*, vol. 30, 2006, pp. 1392–9.

Société royale de médecine, *Nouveau plan de constitution pour la médecine en France présenté à l'Assemblée nationale par la Société royale de médecine*, Paris, 1790.

Summerfield, Carol and Mary Elizabeth Devine, *International Dictionary of University Histories*, Chicago, Fitzroy Dearborn Publishers, 1998.

Sutherland, Donald, 'Etude en Cas: le comité de surveillance d'Aubagne', *Rives nord-méditerranéenesutherland*. http://rives.revues.org/574. doi: 10.4000/rives.574.

Sutherland, Donald, *Murder in Aubagne: Lynching, Law, and Justice during the French Revolution*, Cambridge, Cambridge University Press, 2009.

Vess, David M., 'The collapse and revival of medical education in France: A consequence of revolution and war, 1789–1795', *History of Education Quarterly*, vol. 7, no. 1, Spring, 1967, pp. 71–92.

Wikipedia, *Liste des membres de la Convention nationale par département*. Downloaded 19.11.2018.

7   Ramel and the Military

The record of Ramel's involvement with the French military is fragmented and incomplete. As already discussed, Ramel went to Minorca in 1782/83 a site of previous military conflict.

France started a series of wars in Europe in 1792, and it became apparent that there was a shortage of medical personnel in the military. At the end of 1792 there were only around 1,400 military physicians and surgeons.[1] According to Sir Francis d'Ivernois at this time, "the ravages of epidemic diseases of the military hospitals, which carried off the sick and convalescents, but most of the experienced physicians and surgeons".[2] In a decree dated 1 August 1793, the National Convention required all medical pesonnel, physicians, surgeons, pharmacists, and *officiers de santé* between the ages of 18 and 40 to report to the French Ministry of War.[3] There had been "a huge loss of medically-trained personnel serving with the army".[4] A result of this decree by the end of 1794 numbers had been lifted to 9,000–10,000.[5] Ramel was just too old to be caught by this decree, but that would not have prevented him from volunteering his services. The precise dates of his service are unclear: most probably they were 1793–95; however, there may be some overlap into other years. This decree set out the information, which had to be supplied when an individual was being brought into the army medical service. In turn, approval was in the hands of the *Conseil de santé*, a committee of army and naval personnel. Later that month a mass levée was decreed by the National Convention, which ostensibly conscrpted all French individuals to serve the nation.[6] Avoidance of the call up and desertion were signifivant problems for the military.[7] The extent to which this applied to medical practitioners is unknown; however, examples of avoidance by two doctors are detailed later.[8]

Ramel consistently used the title of *Officier de santé* until he died. *Officier de santé* was a term used for surgeons, pharmacists, and physicians given temporary commissions. Such individuals were not carreer soldiers, and at the end of wars or particular campaigns their status terminated and they were not entitled to a pension.

Ramel's first recorded direct involvement with the military came in 1793, when he stated that he was at the seige of Toulon, which took place between 18 September and 18 December of that year.[9] At this stage he appears to be acting on a voluntary basis. Between 1792 and 1793, a bitter and often violent dispute, raged in the naval port of Toulon (some 50 km from Aubagne and some 35 from La Ciotat) between rival local factions.[10] It came to a head when the local administration allowed a British fleet under the command of Admiral Hood (1724–1816) to take effective control of the naval base. A Republican army arrived from Lyon and based above the city, engaged in a seige, which ultimatly led to the withdrawal of the British force. Given Ramel's Republican sympathies, it is almost certain that he was on the side of the beseigers. The British and Spanish forces were finally ejected in December 1793. By a decree of 24 December 1793, the name of Toulon was changed, as was said at the time, to *"Le nom infâme de Toulon est supprimé. Cette commune portera désormais le nom de Port-la-Montagne"*.[11] Ramel used the name *Port de la Montagne*. His role was described as that of *médecin vacantes*, in effect a locum, and that he tended the sick during the siege.[12]

Napolean Bonaparte, then a captain of artillery, played a significant role in retaking Toulon for the Revolutionary government. This may have been significant for Ramel as Bonapart was to impact on his later life.[13] Ramel joined in as a physician and importantly would have come in contact with Napoleon. During the conflict Napoleon was injured in the thigh by a British soldier; it is possible that he was treated by Ramel. At this time Ramel was largely resident in La Ciotat, and Napoleon corresponded on a number of occasions with the authorities there, including:

> I require you citizens, to strip at once the sun-roof of the chapel (the dome of the Blue Penitents) to have the lead to make bullets; do not forget any of the measures that you can take to procure for us a great quantity of lead. You have a foundry at La Ciotat which is only working a little. It is necessary that you don't want it to stop for an instant; provide some intelligent workers to assist and to learn that trade which is very easy. Let me know me the quantity of bullets that it produces in 24 hours; it is necessary that the furnace is running day and night.[14]

Napoleon was evidently well informed about La Ciotat, and it is possible that Ramel was his source of information. Napoleon used the term *balle*, bullet, but perhaps as an artillery officer he wanted cannon balls, which were normally made of iron.

The records relating to Ramel held by the French Ministry of Defence are limited and not always clearly dated. The earliest is a note of 20 November 1793, in the name of Gautier, Adjutant to the Minister for War, addressed to Citoyen Ramel, Deputy of the Department of the Aude at the National Convention.[15] This Citoyen Ramel was *Dominique-Vincent Ramel-Nogaret (1760–1829) who was unrelated to Ramel le fils*. Marked "Ramel and 2nd Division, 3rd Section, hôpitaux militaire no. 46", it opens with the remark that the ministry has received Ramel de Nogaret's letter of 9 November 1793 and that from Bernadin Ramel le fils. Ramel de Nogaret wrote that Ramel's letter had been passed to the *Conseil de Santé*, but pointing out that more information is required to justify Ramel's standing as a physician, without which he cannot obtain a place.

Ramel wrote to Ramel de Nogaret on 8 February 1794, when he was at La Ciotat, saying that it was two months since he had written, evidently not having received a response. In the interim period he had been working in the military hospitals. He was enclosing a *certificat de civisme* – a republican document showing a person to be of good behaviour and politically orthodox, an attestation from the Aubagne hospital, an attestation from the administration of the hospital at La Ciotat where he had worked gratis during the billeting of three battalions, and a list of his publications. Whilst he refers to his experience in hospitals at Aubagne and La Ciotat, he does not mention his degree from Aix-en-Provence. Neither does he mention his time in La Calle or his visit to Minorca. His publications would have evidenced his work at La Calle and Minorca though not obvious from just a listing. He added a footnote that he had served as a "*médecin vacantes*" at the *Port de la montagne* (Toulon); in effect he had been a locum.[16]

The Adjutant 1st division, 3rd section military hospital replied to this letter 14 March 1794. The hand-writing of this individual appears different to the Adjutant Gautier, noting that Ramel has complied with the requirements of the law of the 1 August and has sent to the *Conseil de santé* Ramel's attestations and capacities. He had written the *Conseil* to remind him of the request to serve in the military hospitals of the Republic. On this basis, it would appear that Ramel had not been formally accepted as an *Officier de santé* in the army at that time.

A further signed and detailed document is a pro-forma used for the records of an *officier de santé*. This required details laid out in the *Décret de la Convention Nationale du première août 1793*: name, age, previous occupation, father's occupation, and places of birth and residence, and, additionally on this form, whether the individual was a physician, surgeon, or pharmacist. Ramel is described as a physician. Whilst it recorded that Ramel was a resident of La Ciotat, it stated that at the time he was a physician in *l'Armée d'Italie* in Oneille. It appears to be dated 15 messidor l'an 2 (3 July 1794) and was certified by members of *"la comité révolutionaire de France"* in Oneille.[17] The other information this document provided was that Ramel served in La Ciotat hospital gratuitously during the Revolution. Furthermore it stated that he was involved with the sick during the siege of *Port de la Montagne*. Much of this was a reiteration of what Ramel had himself written in his letter referred to above.

The problem with this form is ascertaining its date; it has been marked *15 messidor an 2* (3 July 1794), but the *15 messidor* has been struck out. If by accident, and that appears as possibly the case, this document probably is a record of his formal acceptance as an *officier de santé*, if it was deliberate, then his formal status is unknown. In a number of his publications Ramel referred to himself as an *officier de santé*, though more often as a *médecin*. He also made reference to serving for three years in the *Armée d'Italie* in a number of his publications. In *Sur L'Influence des marais et des étangs*, he stated that "I was for three years *'Médecin de l'Armée d'Italie'*".[18] In the same work, he claimed that he had practiced medicine for three years in the most "considerable" hospitals of the Army of Italy and at others and hospices in Toulon, Nice, and Oneille.[19] Desgenettes, his superior officer at the time, stated that Ramel was at Oneille.[20] However, Desgenettes was not particularly impressed by Ramel's discipline, remarking that "Ramel... was always meddling in political affairs, disappeared one moment, went to hide in the Genoan territory, making himself suspect to being an *émigré* and endangering me; because I appeared to have ignored the fact".[21] Just what Ramel meant by "the most considerable hospitals" he did not elaborate on; however, Desgenettes described the military hospitals at Nice, Villefranche, and Monaco in similar terms.[22] He claimed the Monaco hospital as able to comfortably accomodate 500 patients. Ramel did not specifically refer to being in Antibes although he evidently was there.[23] Desgenettes went to Italy in February 1793 and in January 1794 took over from Ramel in Antibes where they first met.[24]

Desgenettes said of Ramel that he was "around 50", of stocky build, his ample head always firmly fixed between his very round shoulders. Perhaps he looked older than his years, as at this time, he was only 42 years old. Desgenettes continued his description: "The facial expression of Ramel, on which was portayed the strength of his mind and a very disturbed character, expressed moreover a self-satisfaction which went as far as a disdain for others".[25]

Desgenettes wrote:

> By chance the first person to whom I spoke at Antibes was Ramel, who I mistook for the owner of a *cabaret borgne*[26], which offended him greatly... Preparation for dinner took a little long, and the hostess in order to keep me patient, made conversation with me. She was a large, young and beautiful blond, which is rare in Provence, and very gentle, which also is not very common. 'Monsieur, she said to me, so you are going to be our new doctor? That's very good.' Hmm, I replied, what do you know about this...? We have, she replied, a veritable villain of a doctor, who is proud, avaricious, and only hangs out with troublemakers like himself.' Dr Ramel I asked?, Yes, that is of whom I speak and to think he replaced such a good man, who would not be dead, if he had looked after himself better.[27]

There followed a brief discussion of Ramel's predecessor, Dr Manuel de Barcelonnette,[28] followed by a description of the meal which was served.

Ramel had returned in a bad humour, and learning a little late who I was or what I had come to do, faced up to the tavern in order to greet me. They made him wait until Desgenettes had finished his coffee. Entering, Ramel said:

> You will do better than me in this place, I see by the way they pampered you on arrival. I leave unhappy and will have no regret. Antibes offers only a cold population, uncivil and very introverted. – Perhaps dear friend, that the Antbois in their turn find you too hot and put too high a price on your services? – There is perhaps something in that – Besides, I am going, if you find it good, take with your coffee a small glass of liquor; it is excellent in this house, but very dear... If you should happen at Aubagne, and that I am there, I will be delighted to return kindness with kindness.[29]

From this brief record of the encounter between Ramel and Desgenettes, it is reasonable to conclude that Ramel had not established a good relationship with at least some of the Antbois. It is equally clear that Ramel was happy to be leaving the town. What is not clarified is what happened after he left Antibes. The above conversation took place in January or February 1794. As will be shown later, in November of that year, Ramel was in Oneille, so he had not at that stage returned to La Ciotat in the western Var.

There is a further document marked 2nd Division, 3rd Section, hôpital militaire no. 46 from Paul Gautier, the Adjutant General in the *Armée d'Italie* dated 13 March 1794 to the Ministry of War supporting Ramel's application.[30] The remaining documents cannot be interpreted or their relevance investigated, they constitute eight small pages with illegible signatures and dates and no text.

Ramel was specific about serving in the *Armée d'Italie*. The structure of the French army changed in the 1790s. In April 1792 *l'Armée du midi* was created only to be split in October of that year into *l'Armée des Alpes*, *l'Armée des Pyrénées*, and *l'Armée d'Italie*; a month later, the latter was split into *l'Armée d'Italie* and *l'Armée de Savoie*.[31] It was the *l'Armée d'Italie* with which Ramel stated he served those three years.[32] He specifically stated that he had been in the *Armée d'Italie* since 1793. The precise dates of his military service are not clear, but probably covered the period 1793–95. Thus, it would appear that this aspect of his military service commenced immediately after the siege of Toulon described previously.

Physicians did not have front line roles, surgeons were at the battle front. Indeed it has been claimed by Hudon and Keel that in times of war the master-surgeon was on equal standing with the physician.[33] In civilian life the physician was regarded as the superior of a surgeon, by education and social standing. When Dominique Jean Larry (1766–1842) introduced his mobile ambulances they were manned by surgeons and assistants whose job it was to return injured soldiers to a field hospital, then on to a more permanent hospital if necessary.

In military hospitals physicians and surgeons of comparable standing were paid the same.[34] The annual rates of pay ranged from a chief physician/surgeon at 2,000 livres down; physicians and surgeon-majors of the lowest order receiving 600 livres.[35] By way of comparison, the surgeon-major at La Calle was paid 500 livres.[36] The rates for supernumeries is unknown.The *Ordonnance du roi* of 1781 only stated that they were under the direction of military physicans dedicated to a military hospital but could take over in the absence of the latter.[37] It was mainly in hospitals that a physician might be found. Not only were there physical casualties of war, most of which would have required surgical attention, but disease, particularly those of a feverous nature. Desgenettes has detailed many of the varied illnesses for which the soldiers in the Armée d'Italie were hospitalized.[38] This was a constant cause of soldiers being unfit to fight. Probably the most important work on military medicine of the period was written by the Scottish physician Sir John Pringle (1707–82), whom Ramel quoted on various occasions.[39] The general requirements for the operation and supplying of military hospitals was set out in some detail in a regulation of 1781.[40] However, when the Revolution came conditions in these hospitals were often found to be unsatisfactory, and considerable effort was made to improve them.[41] In a discourse aimed at improving military hospitals, *premier médecin des campes et armées du Roi*, Jean-François Coste (1741–1810) laid down the standing and role of a physician in such establishments.[42]

Ramel's application to be recognized as an *officier de santé* leaves some unanswered questions. As he was already a *médecin*, a physician, why did he want such recognition? Was it so that he had official standing in the army – this term had been used under the *ancien régime* to designate members of the medical corps? On the other hand, it was a term adopted under the Revolution, at one point at least, to be applied to anybody, formally qualified or not, who practiced healing. After 1803, *officier de santé* was applied only to "second class" practitioners. Curiously in this context, Ramel refered to many times giving instructions to *officiers de santé* in the *Armée d'Italie* who were answerable to him, indicating that his was a position superior to that of these *officier de santé*.[43] Did Ramel's use of the term in some way reflect his concern that his degree in medicine was not from one of the three schools of medicine, Paris, Montpellier, and Strasbourg established in 1794? We will never know, what is certain, is that Ramel continued to use both terms *officier de santé* and *médecin* up until his death.[44]

That Ramel was working in Antibes has already been discussed. It would have been around the same time, perhaps a little earlier, that he was based in Nice.This town, which had been part of the Kingdom of Sardinia, was taken by *l'Armée d'Italie*, almost without combat in September 1792.[45] It is noticeable that the official military records including Ramel's letter to the Ministry of War, makes no mention of serving in Nice. Once again Ramel may have had contact with or been known to Napoleon. The dates that Ramel may have been in Nice are unknown, but probably 1794 as it was from here that the *armée* moved to take Oneille where Ramel served. Napoleon, now a brigadier general, was involved in taking Nice and was briefly imprisoned there in 1794. The literature is conflicting as to where and why this took place. According to J.W. Robertson, Napoleon was arrested and held in Nice, being charged with being a terrorist.[46] Arnault and Pancoucke stated Napoleon was imprisoned for refusing to allow his artillery horses to be redeployed.[47] The more likely truth is that he was arrested for his connection to Robespierre, who had been arrested and subsequently executed; Napoleon was incarcerated in the Chateau d'Antibes on the grounds of treason, having made a secret visit to Genoa and was only held for two weeks.[48]

It is almost certain that after Nice, Ramel found himself in Oneille, now known as Oneglia, which was a small principality in the Republic of Genoa.[49] On 19 April 1794, with Napoleon in charge of the artillery, the town was taken. Ramel was certainly in Oneille in November 1794.[50,51] A major task of the physician was to deal with epidemics of fever. It was reported on 1 September 1794 that at the hospital at Onielle there were continuously 700–800 fever cases, and the physicians were very busy.[52] Jean-François Coste in calculating the cost of military hospitals reckoned on a soldier being in such establishments for 46 days.[53] As Ramel was at this hospital in 1794 he would have been involved in treating these feverous patients.

Ramel makes reference to dealing with malignant fevers at various locations:

> Maligne fevers, characterized by purple spots and gangrenous eruptions are generally contagious. We have made this observation... in the Aubagne hospital,... that of la Ciotat,... in that of the *Compagnie d'Afrique* [La Calle] and finally in the principle hospices of the *Armée d'Italie*.[54]

In order to deal with what were described as "infectious miasmas" hospitals were described by Ramel as being disinfected by fumigating with "sulphuric and hydrochloric acids".[55] This did not mean that they sprayed mineral acids around; in practice the acids were used in conjunction with various salts to create disinfecting fumes.[56] Just when, and under what circumstances, Ramel ceased his involvment with the military is not recorded. It is unlikely that he received a pension after such a short period of service. How sucessful he was in a military role cannot be discerned from the records.there is evidence to suggest that he failed to become popular with the local population in towns in which he was based. It would appear that he resumed his medical practice in La Ciotat around 1794, but he may have been engaged in military hospitals there.

Notes

1 Jacques Sandeau, 'La santé aux armées. L'organisation du service et les hôpitaux. Grandes figures et dures réalités', *Revue du Souvenir napoléonien*, vol. 450, January 2004, p. 20.
2 Francis d'Ivernois, *Historical and Political Survey of the Losses Sustained by the French Nation in Population, Agriculture, Colonies, Manufactures and Commerce in Consequence of the Revolution and the Present War*, London, J. Wright, 1799, p. 7.
3 *Decret de la Convention Nationale du première août 1793, l'an second de la République Français qui met à la réquisition du Ministre de la Guerre les officiers de santé, pharmaciens, chirurgiens et Médecins depuis dix-huit ans jusq' à quarante*, Paris, Ministre de la Guerre, 1793.
4 Maurice Crossland, 'The *Officiers de Santé* of the French Revolution: A case study in the changing language of medicine', *Medical History*, vol. 48, no. 2, 2004, p. 233.
5 Sandeau, p. 20.
6 See Wikipedia, 'Levée en Masse', Downloaded 19.11.2018. 'From this moment until such time as its enemies shall have been driven from the soil of the Republic, all Frenchmen are in permanent requisition for the services of the armies. The young men shall fight; the married men shall forge arms and transport provisions; the women shall make tents and clothes and shall serve in the hospitals; the children shall turn old lint into linen; the old men shall betake themselves to the public squares in order to arouse the courage of the warriors and preach hatred of kings and the unity of the Republic.'
7 See Alan Forrest, *Conscripts and Deserters: The Army and French Society during the Revolution and Empire*, Oxford, Oxford University Press, 1989.
8 See p. 86 below.
9 Vincennes, 'The application form'.
10 For a description of this affair see M.H. Crook, 'Federalism and the French revolution: The revolt of Toulon in 1793'. *History*, vol. 65, no. 215, 1980, pp. 383–97; and Willian S, Cormack and Michael Sydenham, 'Counter Revolution? Toulon 1793', *History Today*, vol. 37, 10 October 1987, pp. 49–55.
11 Espace de ressources pédagogiques des Archives du Var, Service educatif des Archives départementales du Var, p. 3. www.archives.var.fr, Accessed 2.2.2015.
12 Letter to Ramel de Nogaret, 8 February 1784.
13 See pp. 93–4 below on mayorality.

14 Marius Deidier, *La Ciotat pendant la période révolutionnaire 1789–95*, La Ciotat, Imprimerie du Vieux Moulin, 1961, p. 58.

15 Ministère de la Défense, Gautier letter of 20 Nov. 1793 to *Dominique-Vincent Ramel. 30 Brumaire, an ii.*

16 Vincennes, Letter to Ramel de Nogaret, 8 February 1784.

17 Vincennes, 'The proforma'.

18 Marie-François-Bernadin Ramel, *De L'Influence des marais et des étangs sur la santé de l'homme*, Marseille, Imprimeure-Libraire de J. Mossy, An X [1801/1802], p. 75.

19 Ibid., p. 79.

20 Desgenettes, *Souvenirs de la fin du XVIIIe siècle*, p. 394.

21 Ibid., p. 394.fn. 1.

22 René Nicolas Dufriche Desgenettes, *Notes pour servir à l'histoire de l'armée d'Italie Recueilles par R Desgenettes*, n.d., Paris, Panckoucke, p. 10.

23 René Nicolas Dufriche Desgenettes, *Souvenirs de la fin du XVIIIe siècle et du commencement du XIXe ou mémoires du R.D.G.* 2 vols., Paris, chez Firmin Didot Frères Libraires, 1836, pp. 316–21.

24 Ibid., pp. 315.

25 Ibid., pp. 316.

26 *Cabaret borgne*, is described in contemporary dictionaries as a bad small tavern little frequented by respectable people.

27 Desgenettes, *Souvenirs de la fin du XVIIIe siècle*, pp. 316–17.

28 This doctor is not to be confused with the Jacques-Antoine Manuel de Barcelonnette (1775–1827) who served in the *Armée d'Italie* at this time, but was not a physician.

29 Desgenettes, *Souvenirs de la fin du XVIIIe siècle*, pp. 319–20.

30 Vincennes, Gautier letter of 14 March 1794. I have been unable to identify the location of hospital 46.

31 Michel Peronnet, 'Naissance du Midi pendant la revolution', *Hystorika Studia Metodologiczne*, Special issue, 2012, p. 138.

32 Ramel, *De L'Influence des marais*, p. 133.

33 Philippe Hudon and Othmar Keel, 'La pratique clinique et thérapeutique dans les armées Français: Le développement de la collaboration entre les médecins, chirurgiens et pharmaciens (1750–1800)', in Olivier Faure (ed.) *Les Thérapeutiques: savoirs et usages*, Lyon, Collection Fondation Marcel Merieux, 1999, p. 209.

34 See Louis XVI, *Ordonnance du roi, portant les règlements générale concernant les hôpitaux militaires*, Paris, n.p., du 2 May 1781, pp. 101–2.

35 Louis XVI, *Ordonnance du roi*, pp. 101–2.

36 Paul Masson, *Histoire des établissements et du commerce Français dans l'a Afrique Barbaresque (1560–1793)*, Paris, Libraire Hachette, 1903, p. 430.

37 Louis XVI, *Ordonnance du roi*, pp. 97 and 140.

38 Desgenettes, *Notes pour servir à l'Histoire de l'armée.*

39 (Sir) John Pringle, *Observations on the Diseases of the Army, in Camp and Garrison. In Three Parts. With an Appendix, Containing Some Papers of Experiments, Read at Several Meetings of the Royal Society*, 2nd edn, corr. and enl., London, A. Millar and D. Wilson, 1752.

40 Louis XVI, *Ordonnance du roi.*

41 See Alan A. Forrest, *The Soldiers of the French Revolution*, Durham, Duke University Press, 1990, pp. 144–150.

42 Jean-François Coste, *Du Service hôpitaux militaires*, Paris, chez Croullebois, 1790, pp. 85–97.

43 Ramel, *De L'Influence des marais*, p. 75.

44 For a fuller discussion the term officier de santé see Robert Heller, 'Officiers de santé: The second-class doctors of nineteenth-century France', *Medical History*, vol. 22, 1978, pp. 25–43. doi:10.1017/S00257 27300031732 and Maurice Crosland, 'The *Officiers de Santé* of the French Revolution: A case study in the changing language of medicine', *Medical History*, vol. 48, no. 2, 2004, pp. 229–44.

45 See Gilles Candella, *L'Armée d'Italie: Nice 1792–1796*, Nice, Serre Éditeur, 2000, p. 14.

46 J. W. Robertson, *The Life and Campaigns of Napoleon Bonaparte: From His Birth Down to His Departure for St. Helena*, Newcastle upon Tyne, Mackenzie and Kent, 1815, p. 21.

47 M.A. Arnault and C.L.F. Pancoucke, *Life and Campaigns of Napoleon Bonaparte Giving an Account of All His Engagements from the Siege of Toulon to the Battle of Waterloo*, Trans from the French, two volumes in one, New Edition, Philadelphia, Porter and Coates, n.d., vol. 1, p. 28. https://archive.org/details/lifecampaignsofn00arna, Accessed 20.1. 2015.

48 David G. Chandler, *The Campaigns of Napoleon*, New York, Scribner 1966, p. 34.

49 Encyclopedia Britannica, www.britannica.com/EBchecked/topic/429122/ Oneglia

50 The Proforma.

51 Candella, pp. 107–8.

52 Ibid., p. 171.

53 Jean François Coste, *Du Service hôpitaux militaires*, p. 239.

54 Ramel, *De L'Influence des marais*, p. 170.

55 Ibid., p. 309.

56 For a description of the disinfection processes see Louis-Bernard Guyton de Morveau, (1737–1816), *Traité des moyens de désinfecter l'air, de prévenir la contagion, et d'en arrêter les progres*, Paris, Chez Bernard, libraire de l'Ecole polytechnique, 1801. In 1794, on the instruction of the *Comité de Santé*, the Ministry of War required all military hospitals to be fumigated, pp. 20–1, Porter and Coates, n.d., https://archive. org/details/lifecampaignsofn00arna, Accessed 09.01.2017.

Bibliography

Arnault, M.A., and C.L.F. Pancoucke, *Life and Campaigns of Napoleon Bonaparte Giving an Account of All His Engagements from the Siege of Toulon to the Battle of Waterloo*, Trans from the French, two volumes in one, New Edition, Philadelphia, Porter and Coates, n.d., https://archive. org/details/lifecampaignsofn00arna, Accessed 9.1.2017.

Candella, Gilles, *L'Armée d'Italie: Nice 1792–1796*, Nice, Serre Éditeur, 2000.

Chandler, David C., *The Campaigns of Napoleon*, New York, Scribner, 1966.

Cormack, William S. and Michael Sydenham, 'Counter revolution? Toulon 1793', *History Today*, vol. 37, 10 October 1987, pp. 49–55.

Coste, Jean-François, *Du Service hôpitaux militaires*, Paris, chez Croullebois, 1790.

Crook, M.H. 'Federalism and the French Revolution: The Revolt of Toulon in 1793', *History*, vol. 65, no. 215, 1980, pp. 383–97.

Crosland, Maurice, 'The *Officiers de Santé* of the French revolution: A case study in the changing language of medicine', *Medical History*, vol. 48, no. 2, 2004, pp. 229–44.

Decret de la Convention Nationale du première août 1793, l'an second de la République Français qui met à la réquisition du Ministre de la Guerre les officiers de santé, pharmaciens, chirurgiens et Médecins depuis dix-huit ans jusq' à quarante, Paris, Ministre de la Guerre, 1793.

Deidier, Marius., *La Ciotat pendant la période révolutionnaire 1789–95*, La Ciotat, Imprimerie du Vieux Moulin, 1961.

Desgenettes, René-Nicolas Dufriche, *Notes pour servir à l'histoire de l'armée d'Italie, recueilles par R Desgenettes*, Paris, Panckoucke, n.d.

Desgenettes, René-Nicolas Dufriche, *Souvenirs de la fin du XVIIIe siècle et du commencement du XIXe ou mémoires du R.D.G.* 2 vols., Paris, chez Firmin Didot Frères Libraires, 1836.

d'Ivernois, Sir Francis, *Historical and Political Survey of the Losses Sustained by the French Nation in Population, Agriculture, Colonies, Manufactures and Commerce in Consequence of the Revolution and the Present War*, London, J. Wright, 1799.

Encyclopaedia Britannica, www.britannica.com/EBchecked/topic/429122/ Oneglia, Accessed 22.11.2016.

Espace de ressources pédagogiques des Archives du Var, Service educatif des.

Forrest, Alan A., *Conscripts and Deserters: The Army and French Society during the Revolution and Empire*, Oxford, Oxford University Press, 1989.

Forrest, Alan A., *The Soldiers of the French Revolution*, Durham, Duke University Press, 1990.

Guyton de Morveau, Louis-Bernard, 1737–1816, *Traité des moyens de désinfecter l'air, de prévenir la contagion, et d'en arrêter les progres*, Paris, chez Bernard, libraire de l'Ecole polytechnique, 1801.

Heller, Robert, 'Officiers de Santé: The second-class doctors of nineteenth-century France', *Medical History*, vol. 22, no. 1, 1978, pp. 25–43.

Hudon, Philippe and Othmar Keel, 'La pratique clinique et thérapeutique dans les armées Français: Le développement de la collaboration entre les médecins, chirurgiens et pharmaciens (1750–1800)', in Olivier Faure (ed.) *Les Thérapeutiques: savoirs et usages*, Lyon, Collection Fondation Marcel Merieux, 1999, pp. 209–21.

Louis XVI, *Ordonnance du roi, portant les règlements générale concernant les hôpitaux militaires*, du 2 May 1781, Paris, n.p.

Masson, Paul, *Histoire des établissements et du commerce Français dans l'a Afrique Barbaresque (1560–1793)*, Paris, Libraire Hachette, 1903.

Perronet, Michel, 'Naissance du Midi', in Jean Sentou (ed.) *Révolution et contre-révolution dans la France du midi 1789–1799*, Toulouse, Presses universitaires du Mirail, 1991, pp. 25–6.

Pringle, (Sir) John, *Observations on the Diseases of the Army, in Camp and Garrison. In Three Parts. With an Appendix, Containing Some Papers of Experiments, Read at Several Meetings of the Royal Society, 2nd edn, corr. and enl.*, London, A. Millar and D. Wilson, 1752.

Ramel, Marie-François-Bernadin, *De L'Influence des marais et des étangs sur la santé de l'homme*, Marseille, Imprimeure-Libraire de J. Mossy, An X [1801/1802].

Robertson, J.W., *The Life and Campaigns of Napoleon Bonaparte: From His Birth Down to His Departure for St. Helena*, Newcastle upon Tyne, Mackenzie and Kent, 1815.

Sandeau, Jacques, 'La santé aux armées. L'organisation du service et les hôpitaux. Grandes figures et dures réalités', *Revue du Souvenir napoléonien*, vol. 450, January 2004, pp. 19–27.

Service historique de la défense centre historique des archives, Vincennes:
Gautier letter of 14 March 1794.
Gautier letter of 20 November 1793.
Letter to Ramel de Nogaret, 8 February 1784.
Commission de Sante, Officier de Santé proforma for Ramel dated 15 July 1793.
'The application form'.

Wikipedia, 'Levée en Masse', Downloaded 19.11.2018.

8   Civilian Life in La Ciotat

According to Louis Barthélemy, Ramel had departed Aubagne in 1789 or 1790 to the nearby town of La Ciotat where he established a medical practice.[1] However as noted previously, his military records show him as being a resident of La Ciotat since 1786. It is possible that he also maintained an office in Aubagne as he refers to a case in which he saw a man *"à mon cabinet ... à Aubagne"* in November 1801.[2] It is evident that at some stage he reverted to his daily practice as a physician, but the archives do not indicate exactly when this occurred (Figure 8.1).

Ramel was divorced, although neither the precise date nor whether he divorced Anne-Rose-Félicité Lieutard or she divorced him is known. Divorce had not been permitted under the *ancien régime* but was legalized by the National Assembly on 20 September 1792.[3] A number of grounds for obtaining a divorce were listed in the legislation, but the most significant, and probable in Ramel's case, was either abandonment for at least two years or prolonged absence without news for five years.[4] It seems likely that Mme. Lieutard divorced him on the basis of his absence during the period he was serving in the army. A one-year wait was required after divorce before re-marriage was permitted.[5] According to an historian of the French Revolution, many more women divorced their husbands than the other way around.[6] Ramel married a second time, to Claire-Marguerite Bienvenu by whom he had one child, Paul Bernadin Ramel (1795–1857).[7] Assuming Paul was born in wedlock, Ramel's divorce would have been between 1792 and 1794, and this second marriage was between 1794 and 1795.

As previously noted, Ramel was a member of the *Société royale de l'académie d'Arras*. Abbé Louis Berthe has studied the departmental archives of the Pas de Calais and has extracted records of Ramel's involvement in the meetings of the provincial assemblies of Artois in 1787–88. It seems odd that Ramel should have been be

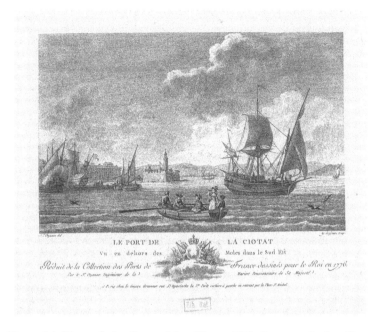

Figure 8.1 View of the Port of La Ciotat 1776. Le *port de La Ciotat* vu en dehors des môles dans le sud est / N[icolas] Ozanne *del*[ineavit]; Y. Le Gouaz sculp[sit] --1776-- cartes. fr/ark:/12148/ btv1b531431847. Courtesy: Bibliothèque nationale de France.

involved in the affairs of a region so far from his home base, but it was in this context that in 1789 he attended meetings of *Les États d'Artois*. *Les États d'Artois* originated in the fourteenth century and was charged with voting on taxes imposed by the King.[8] In effect there was disputation between the nobles and clergy claiming privilege in this matter, and the peasants who claimed common rights to the use of areas for animal pasturage.[9] *L'États* composition consisted of representatives of the clergy, the nobles, and a number of gentlemen. In the latter part of the eighteenth century it became concerned with the administration and jurisdiction of the *marais* in the area.[10] One can only surmise that Ramel became involved in some way recognising his expertise on the topic of marshy land. However, he went beyond that topic, expressing his view on the broader issue of the structure of representational bodies in France, as reported by Berthe, Ramel addressed *Les États d'Artois* thus:

Your provincial assemblies are finally ended: I congratulate you very sincerely. Knowing your love for the work, the lively interest that I take in your well-being makes me learn with pleasure that this job where you are not sparing yourself is finally completed. Ours, after many debates on the precedents and other trifles of this nature, are also coming to an end. Instead of the 300,000 livres voted by your province, ours has generously offered 900,000. I do not disguise also that in spite of the good will of the government, I regard our assemblies as again being very unsound. The wise intention of the King, is, one says, to establish a perfect equality in the voices of the third estate and those of the nobility and of the clergy, reunited together. Consequently, there will be in our assemblies (perhaps also in yours) many deputies of the third estate that will not have sided with the clergy and the nobility. This alleged equality will always incline towards the balance on the side of the clergy or the nobility in all major affaires. Ah! How, you will ask me? Because, among the deputies of the third estate, there will always be, 3, 4, 10, nobles, parents, friends of the nobility, finally as nobles, always disposed to line up on the side of the nobility. But why, you will ask me again will deputies of the third estate be acting like nobles? Because the deputies of the communities representing the third estate are always the first consuls of the communities and that among the first consuls there are always several nobles. This intrinsic fault of the provincial assemblies of which the third estate complains, with foundation, has not yet been seen without doubt by the beneficent government which they have created, But, it is enough that you have to maintain politics and administration. Do not lose sight that men of letters and some academicians only must take care of the sciences.[11]

Berthe added "Doctor Ramel did not come back to this subject. Did he not say in good faith everything that he was thinking at that time"?[12] As to the 9,000 livres which Ramel referred to, this presumably was the sum raised by his own regional *Les États de Provence*, an organization also supressed in 1789.

Returning attention to La Ciotat, the Revolution took hold there in 1789. From January to March there were riots across the Var. At La Ciotat there were riots on 27 March, mainly over taxes and the price of wheat and vegetables. In 1790, André Toussaint Besson became the mayor, but this led to much disputation between the various pro- and anti-revolutionary factions in the town. In 1798 Ramel was appointed secretary to the municipal council.[13] By 1800, however, the Revolution had run out of steam, and on 11 May that year, Ramel was appointed mayor of the town, by Napoleon, who was now First Consul of the Republic. Ramel held the post until October 1803, when he was replaced, although he remained on the council.[14] The reason given at the time for losing his position was deteriorating health; however, it may be that Ramel, as a firm adherent to the ideals of the Revolution, ceased to fit with the changing local political scene in the early nineteenth century.[15] Whenever Ramel's name appears in the municipal archives of La Ciotat he is described as an *Officier de santé*, with the exception of his municipally recorded death.

It was concern for the future of his son that Ramel called on the services of César Couret, whose maturity in a crisis during the Revolution noted earlier, had impressed Ramel. Couret in his history of Aubagne recorded that Ramel in 1810 had summoned him, saying:

> I want you know, he said to me, what has been told about you interests me in your position. I entrust to your care the instruction of my only son, persuaded of some wise lessons that you can give to him, I will pay you double that which you ordinarily receive. Here is my library it is for your use. Take today some of the volumes of your choice; I lend them to you for a month; after this time, you return them to me and I will entrust you with some others. Educate yourself my friend, knowledge is the most precious of treasures. If in your reading some passage bothers you, come to me to find out, I would be at your service, use my very weak knowledge.[16]

At this time Couret was 28 years old. Ramel's son Paul would have been 15 years old, and one can also presume that Ramel had probably realized that he was reaching the end of his life; as he was losing or had lost his sight, he was looking for somebody to guide the boy. How successful Couret was in this task is unknown. When he wrote about this conversation, 1860, Couret described himself as a retired *notaire*. Although he described himself as a graduate of the University of France, to be a *notaire* at that time required no training, one simply had to be able to read and write.[17] As was shown earlier, Ramel had been much impressed by Couret's handling of a difficult family crisis during the Revolution despite Couret's youth. Given that it is evident that Paul did not follow the family tradition into medicine, one can reasonably conclude that to be of value to Couret in educating the boy, Ramel's collection of books must have had a much wider scope than just medical texts. This was a common feature of physicians' libraries at the time.

The date and time of Ramel's death is recorded in the La Ciotat municipal records as occurring on 7 January 1811 at four o'clock in the afternoon, aged 62, and describes him as a *"docteur en Medicine"*.[18] The municipal record does not state the cause of death. Of the signatories to this record was the current mayor, Mathieu Payar Latour.

Whilst there is no reason to doubt the recorded date of his death, the stated age appears in contradiction to other documented dates. Barthélemy wrote that he died aged 58,[19] and a more likely age was 59.[20] In 1823 the physician Alexis Pujol, who claimed to be a regular correspondent with Ramel, lamented the fact that he was unable to contact him. Evidently his demise had gone unnoticed outside his local community. No eulogy appears to have been written, probably because by the time he died, the *Société royale de médicine* had been supressed, and its successor, the *Société médicine de Paris*, had not started to publish such items. Perhaps the nearest thing to a eulogy came in the form of a *mémoire* written in 1789, probably by Vicq d'Azyr:

> M. Ramel, doctor at Aubagne is distinguished by his zeal, by the acuity of his correspondence, by the new and interesting details that he has communicated, and by the precision with which he has written his observations which he has made over 4 years ... The Society wants to give recognition to M. Ramel, [and] has awarded, in the séance of 1 September 1789, a medal to the value of one gold jeton.[21]

This memoire, written in the context of epilepsy on which Ramel had evidently corresponded, although no record appears to have survived, is praise indeed. What is also unusual is the awarding of the medal. The *Société* frequently awarded prizes to individuals who submitted dissertations on prescribed topics in a competitive manner; this award was made *ad libitum*.

In February 1816, at the early age of 21, Ramel' son Paul, married Marguerite Martine Amelie Daumac of La Ciotat, with his mother consenting.[22] By this time Ramel was already dead, and during the revolutionary period, the age of majority, and hence the ability to marry had been changed to 21 years.[23] At the time of Paul's death he was described as being "a proprietor".[24] Whether this reflected the boy's abilities or interests are an unknown, certainly he did not carry on the family tradition in medicine.

Ramel's final years were spent apparently practising medicine, and, at the same time, taking an active part in local politics. His elevation to the position of mayor gave him some status, although his inability, or more likely unwillingness, to adapt to a changing political environment meant that this was short lived.

Notes

1 Louis Barthélemy, *Histoire d'Aubagne: Chef-lieu de baronnie depuis son origine jusq'en 1789*, 2 vols., Marseille, Lafitte reprints, 1972. (Réimpresion de l'édition de Marseille, 1889), vol. 2, p. 326.

2 Marie-François-Bernadin Ramel, *De L'Influence des marais et des étangs sur la santé de l'homme*, Marseille, Imprimeure-Libraire de J. Mossy, An X [1801/2], fn., p. 128.

3 Chris Roulston, *Narrating Marriage in Eighteenth-Century England and France*, Farnham, Ashgate, 2010, p. 47.

4 Lynn Hunt, 'The unstable boundaries of the French Revolution', in Michelle Perrot, Philippe Ariès, and Georges Duby (eds) *A History of a Private Life From the Fires of Revolution to the Great War*, Cambridge, The Belknap Press of Harvard University Press, 1990, pp. 33–34.

5 Ibid.

6 Suzzane Desan, *The Family on Trial in Revolutionary France*, Berkeley, University of California Press, 2004, p. 95. See also André Burguière, 'La Révolution et la famille', *Annales. Économies, Sociétés, Civilisations*, vol. 46, no. 1, 1991, pp. 151–68. Burguière states that in large towns, around 60% of divorces were initiated by women. p. 160.

7 Barthélemy, vol. 2, p. 327.

8 Les Archives départementales du Pas-de-Calais.

9 Abbé L. Berthe, 'Les Assemblées provinciales et l'opinion publique en 1787–1788', *Revue du Nord*, vol. 46, no. 189, April–June 1966, p. 194.

10 François Filon, *Histoire des États d'Artois depuis leur origine jusqu'à leur suppression en 1789*, Paris, Auguste Durand Libraire, 1861, pp. 92–7; and, L'Abbé Berthe, pp. 185–200.

11 Abbé le Berthe, pp. 194–5. This appears to be a verbatim record of a speech by Ramel 17 February 1788.

12 Berthe, p. 195.

13 Coste, *Les Écrits de la soufrance: La Consultation médicale en France (1550–1825)*, Ceyzérieu, Champ Vallon, 2014, p. 356.

14 Association de la mairie de La Ciotat, www.asso.mairie-laciotat.fr/La-Revolution-et-l-Empire-HISTOIRE-PATRIMOINE/p/3/4266/0/
There are some contradictions regarding the date he ceased to be mayor. The records of mayors of La Ciotat record his tenure as ending in October 1803, yet also shows his successor taking up the position in September 1803; yet another notes him as losing the position in August 1803.

15 Roger Klotz, L'Admiral Ganteaume et les Ciotadens', *Récherches régionales Côte d'Azure et contrées limotrophes*, vol. 5, 2010, n.p.

16 César Couret, *Histoire d'Aubagne: Divisée en trois époques principales*, Aubagne, Michel Baubet, 1860, pp. 108–9.

17 Rauolde de La Groserie (1898), cited in Ezra N, Suleman, *Private Powers and Centralisation in France: The Notaries and the State*, Princeton, Princeton University Press, 2014, p. 132.

18 Archives municipales de la ville de La Ciotat, *Décès 1810–1811*, entry 133.

19 Barthélemy, p. 327.

20 Using all the dates referenced in the found records indicates his age at death to be 59.

21 Pierre-Théophile Barrois (ed.), *Histoire de la Société Royale de Médecine: avec les Mémoires de Médecin: Année MDCCLXXXII et MDCLXXXIII*, Paris, chez Théopile Barrois le jeune, 10 vols., 1779–89, vol. 9, pp. xii–xiii.

22 Archives municipales de la ville de La Ciotat, *Marriages.1816–8*, Entry, 1816/17.

23 Desan, p. 326.

24 Archives municipales de la ville de La Ciotat, *Décès 1828–1829–1839*, entry 133.

Bibliography

Archives municipales de la ville de La Ciotat, *Décès, 1810–1811, 1828–1829–1839; Marriage, 1816–17*.

Association de la mairie de La Ciotat, www.asso.mairie-laciotat.fr/La-Revolution-et-l-Empire-HISTOIRE-PATRIMOINE/p/3/4266/0/

Barrois, Pierre-Théophile (ed.), *Histoire de la Société Royale de Médecine: avec les Mémoires de Médecin: Année MDCCLXXXII et MDCLXXXIII*, Paris, chez Théopile Barrois le jeune, 10 vols., 1779–89.

Barthélemy, Louis, *Histoire d'Aubagne: Chef-lieu de baronnie depuis son origine jusq'en 1789*, 2 vols., Marseille, Lafitte reprints, 1972. (Réimpresion de l'édition de Marseille, 1889.).

Berthe, L., Abbé, 'Les Assemblées provinciales et l'opinion publique en 1787–1788', *Revue du Nord*, vol. 46, no. 189, April–June 1966, pp. 185–200.

Coste, Joël, *Les Écrits de la soufrance: La Consultation médicale en France (1550–1825)*, Ceyzérieu, Champ Vallon, 2014.

Couret, César, *Histoire d'Aubagne: Divisée en trois époques principales*, Aubagne, Michel Baubet, 1860.

Desan, Suzzane, *The Family on Trial in Revolutionary France*, Berkeley, University of California Press, 2004.

Filon, François, *Histoire des Etats d'Artois depuis leur origine jusqu'à leur suppression en 1789*, Paris, Auguste Durand Libraire, 1861.

Hunt, Lynn, 'The unstable boundaries of the French Revolution', in Michelle Perrot, Philippe Ariès, and Georges Duby (eds), *A History of a Private Life From the Fires of Revolution to the Great War*, Cambridge, The Belknap Press of Harvard University Press, 1990, pp. 13–46.

Klotz, Roger, L'Admiral Ganteaume et les Ciotadens', *Récherches régionales Côte d'Azure et contrées limotrophes*, vol. 5, 2010, n.p. Les Archives départementales du Pas-de-Calais.

Ramel, Marie-François-Bernadin, *De L'Influence des marais et des étangs sur la santé de l'homme*, Marseille, Imprimeure-Libraire de J. Mossy, An X [1801/2].

Rauolde de La Groserie (1898), cited in Ezra N, Suleman, *Private Powers and Centralisation in France: The Notaries and the State*, Princeton, Princeton University Press, 2014.

Roulston, Chris, *Narrating Marriage in Eighteenth-Century England and France*, Farnham, Ashgate, 2010.

9 Placing Ramel in His Times

In seeking to be a medical savant, as has been pointed out, Ramel was one of at least 150 correspondents with the *Société royale de medicine*. So in that regard he was far from unique, but there were aspects of his life that set him apart; notably his success in winning awards for his publications, as was his revolutionary fervour. Detailed histories of rural physicians in the early-modern period are uncommon; however, interesting comparisons can be made between Ramel and three roughly contemporary professionals, Pierre-Joseph Amoreux, Esprit Claude François Calvet, and Michel Darluc.

All four were from the Midi, lived and worked in the second half of the eighteenth century, and apart from Darluc, lived through the revolutionary period. There was a tradition of medicine in the Ramel family: his father and grandfather were physicians;[1] Calvet's great-grandfather, grandfather, and father had practiced as apothecaries;[2] Amoreux's grandfather had been a surgeon, and his father had been a physician and natural historian.[3] Darluc, on the other hand, was the son of a master tailor.[4] The early education of Ramel, Calvet, Darluc, and Amoreux was Catholic, and they all went on to obtain doctorates in medicine.

Ramel was born in largely agricultural Aubagne, population around 7,000, although, as noted earlier, he went at a young age to Marseille with its populationin excess of 100,000. Amoreux's birthplace was Beaucaire, a significant river port, with a population of 8,500, which increased hugely during its annual fair. Calvet was born in Avignon, with a population over 26,000, therefore much larger than Aubagne. Avignon differed not only in size, but, technically was, for most of Calvet's life, not part of France, but a papal enclave. Darluc was born in Grimaud, a small town with a population of around 1,100.

Calvet attended Jesuit colleges in Lyon and Avignon.[5] Amoreux was schooled by the *Doctrinaires* in Beaucaire[6], and, as has been shown, Ramel was educated by Oratorians. Darluc went to a *collège de Trinitaires* in the town of Lorgues, some 30 km from Grimaud, where he studied rhetoric, philosophy, and natural history.[7] As shown before, Ramel attended a small medical faculty in Aix-en-Provence; Calvet studied medicine in Avignon, where the medical faculty was also small and not particularly highly regarded, although he furthered his medical studies at the more prestigious schools of Montpellier and Paris.[8] Calvet obtained his doctoral bonnet at Avignon in 1749. Amoreux attended the Medical University in Montpellier. Prior to the Revolution, the University of Medicine in Montpellier was a separate entity to the University of Montpellier, and it was prestigious. Amoreux commenced studying there in 1757, and he obtained an education beyond mere book-based theory.[9] He obtained his doctoral bonnet in 1762.[10]

Like Ramel, Darluc also went to *la collège d'Oratoire* at Marseille. However, it was at this point that his "education" differed from the others. Instead of proceeding to university, Darluc was offered a position in the service of Provençal dignitary Charles-François Bouche (1736–95), with whom he travelled to Italy, Austria Germany, Corsica, and Spain. He was in Barcelona for two years where he entered the medical school before transferring his studies to the University of Aix-en-Provence in 1740–41. After three years, aged 27 years, he completed his thesis and was awarded his doctorate in 1744.[11] At the beginning of 1745 he went to Paris and studied under chemist Guillaume François Ruelle (1703–70) at the *Jardin du Roi* and probably followed other courses at this institution.[12] In 1747, he returned to the town of his birth and ran a medical practice. The precise dates are somewhat contradictory. Collomp states that he practised in Grimaud from 1747 to 1752 but also that he moved to nearby Callian, where he practised medicine from 1750 or 1751 until 1770.[13] Perhaps at some point he worked from both locations.

Amoreux rapidly showed that he was as interested in natural history as in medicine, which was to become increasingly evident through his life, no doubt influenced by his father who was a well-known naturalist.[14] Calvet on the other hand built up a medical practice, almost certainly larger than Ramel managed to achieve. Nonetheless, Calvet became increasingly interested in antiquities, which none of the others did. Laurence Brockliss has described Calvet as a *"bibliophile, antiquare et naturaliste"*.[15] As to travel, Calvet engaged in further medical learning in Paris and Montpellier, whilst Amoreux travelled to Paris on no less than eight occassions during his lifetime. Ramel alone, it appears travelled out of France.

The French Revolution did not affect Darluc as he died before its commencment, the other three were however affected in different ways. Ramel's involvement in the Revolution and the military has been described; Calvet's and Amoreux's experiences and political attitudes to the Revolution were markedly different to Ramel's. Unlike Ramel, Calvet was not of a revolutionary turn of mind. Avignon, despite it not being a part of France when the Revolution broke out, was nonetheless far from free of social disruption, "political turmoil ... soon ingulfed his city".[16] In 1792 Calvet had soldiers billeted in his house, which had been burgled, and he lost some of his antiquarian collection. To avoid the anarchy Calvet stayed away from Avignon for a couple of years before returning and trying to avoid attention. However, in 1794 he was arrested and incarcerated for three months. Brockliss quotes the reason as being "For never having ceased to manifest anti-civic opinions and for being an extremely pronounced aristocrat".[17] Brockliss continues that to safeguard himself from further harrasment, on his release he volunteered his services to the Army of Italy. Eventually he was sucesssful in placating the authorities, and for 400 livres plus allowances per month, he worked in a local hospital treating injured soldiers.[18] This sum appears a lot when compared with the rates laid down im the *Ordinnance du roi* of 1781, referred to earlier. Like Ramel, he was too old to be conscripted, and his decision to cooperate with the authorities was most probably a device to save his neck rather than commitment to the revolutionary cause.[19] However, he continued to play a public role for several years.[20] Brockliss adds, that "[Th]e Revolution left him bitter and suspicious".[21] All this was so different to Ramel's revolutionary and military efforts and attitudes. Calvet worked as a physician until he reached the age of 74.[22]

Amoreux's *Souvenirs ou details historiques* contains little reference to the effects on him of the Revolution.[23] According to Brockliss, he "disliked it [the Revolution], but co-operated with the new authorities",[24] and Amoreux wrote:

Not exercising medicine, I was hoping not to be required to serve in the army at Boulou, or in the hospitals of Perpignan, by order of the representatives of the people, order of the physician in chief etc. These orders were notified to me by the Commissioner of War, Naudin.[25]

He was apparently successful in his efforts to avoid these alternative impositions, having produced documents to show that he no longer practised medicine. Three of the physicians discussed here were notionally at least liable to be dragooned into serving in the army although in theory they were all too old to be conscripted. Ramel was enthusiastic to be a part of the military, Calvet served reluctantly, and Amoreux dodged it completely.

Although Calvet wrote to the *Academié royale de Médicine*, he made far fewer contributions to that body, or to other learned societies, than did Ramel.[26] Brockliss describes his limited output of written material as:

> In his prime he was a hospital physician and a professor of medicine at his local university as well as a doctor with a solid practice. He could only participate in the Republic of Letters in the evening and would never have had the free time to produce a constant stream of essays and pamphlets.[27]

His practice was almost certainly larger than Ramel's.[28] Calvet's main interest outside his medicine was as an antiquarian collector particularly of shells, fossils, and coins.[29] Neither Amoreux, Darluc, nor Ramel had comparable collections.

Amoreux's record of published and unpublished work is remarkable amounting to an incredible 100 books and articles.[30]. Early in his career he threw himself into submitting papers for prizes with gusto.[31] Like Ramel, Amoreux was a corresponding member of the *Société royale de médecine*. According to Brockliss, Amoreux entered essays for which prizes were offered by the *Société* on five occasions; in 1786 he won a third prize on the topic of the geography and medicine around Montpellier, and in 1790, he was awarded a certificate of merit for a memoire on hereditary diseases.[32] These do not compare with Ramel's five medals from the *Societé*; however, these were not all of Amoreux's prize-essay entries; Brockliss lists a number of provincial and Parisian institutions to which he made such submissions.[33] Indeed, Brockliss describes him as obsessive with respect to entering into prize competitions.[34] Undoubtedly, like Ramel, he sought to establish his significance in the Republic of Letters. Not all his papers were on medical topics; his prime interest was agronomy.[35] He also wrote on the historiography of medicine. In all, he published some 13 books and pamphlets.[36] He became the librarian of *La Société royale des sciences de Montpellier.* To the extent that he was a collector, it was to be through his herbarium, consistent with his interest in natural history and agriculture.[37]

All four physicians were associate members of the *Société royale de médicine* in Paris and submitted a number of papers to that organization, although not all were published. Between 1755 and 1764 Amoreux published 12 articles in the *Journal de médecine* on various medical issues, mostly related to matters that arose in the locality where he was working.[38] He corresponded on a number of occasions with Calvet.[39] He was awarded one prize in August 1781, although its value and subject matter are unknown.[40] Darluc wrote many papers on medical topics, particularly on local epidemics, but was best known for *Natural History of Provence* for which the *société royale* awarded a prize, of unknown value, for the first two volumes.[41,42]

Calvet taught anatomy at the Avignon School of Medicine; Darluc was professor of medicine, holding the chair of botany and natural history at Aix-en-Provence. One of his notable achievements was the creation of a botanic garden at the Aix University. It was unusual for such facilities in that it was open to the public.[43] Amoreux avoided formal connection with the Montpellier School of Medicine. However, during the Revolution, he was coerced into the role of professor of natural history at the Montpellier *école centrale*.[44] Ramel had no academic connections during his working life.

Thus, all these four rural physicians looked beyond practicing medicine. Ramel, sought to make a mark in the Republic of Letters, as did Amoreux, though the latter with a broader field of interest. Calvet on the other hand worked asiduously to maintain a circle of enlightenment contacts in a more localized arena. Amoreux and Calvet endeavoured to leave enlightenment legacies, in that both left much of their books and collections to their respective towns.[45] The ultimate fate of Ramel's library is unknown.

Ramel and Amoreux appear to have remained historically obscure until recently. Calvet, on the other hand, has achieved a more permanent standing, largely due to the fact that he donated much of his collection to the municipality of Avignon, which formed the foundation of the well-known Musée Calvet, which remains significant today.

Notes

1 Louis Barthélemy, *Histoire d'Aubagne: Chef-lieu de baronnie depuis son origine jusq'en 1789*, 2 vols., Marseille, Lafitte reprints, 1972. (Réimpresion de l'édition de Marseille, 1889), vol. 2, p. 324.

2 Laurence Brockliss, *Calvet's Web: Enlightenment and the Republic of Letters in Eighteenth-Century France*, Oxford, Oxford University Press, 2002, pp. 22–4.

3 Laurence Brockliss, *From Provincial Savant to Parisian Naturalist*, Oxford, Voltaire Foundation, University of Oxford, 2017, pp. 26–7.

4 Allain Collomp, *Un médecin des lumières: Michel Darluc, naturaliste provençal*, Rennes, Presses universitaires de Rennes, 2011, pp. 27–8.

5 Brockliss, *Calvet's Web*, p. 258.

6 Brockliss, *From Provincial Savant*, p. 117.

7 Collomp, p. 29. The *Trinitaires* were established in Lorgues in 1359. In the eighteenth century they provided education of the young in religion and Latin.

8 Brockliss, *Calvet's Web*, p. 142.

9 Laurence Brockliss and Colin Jones, *The Medical World of Early Modern France*, Oxford, Clarendon Press, 1997, pp. 513–14.

10 Brockliss, *Calvet's Web*, p. 137.

11 Collomp, p. 42.

12 Ibid., p. 43.

13 Collomp, p. 60.

14 Brockliss, *From Provincial Savant*, p. 28.

15 Laurence Brockliss, 'La République des lettres et les médecins en France à la veille de la Révolution: le cas d'Esprit Calvet', *Gesnerus*, vol. 61, 2004, p. 259.

16 Brockliss, *Calvet's Web*, p. 33. Avignon along with the Comtat Venaisin was a Papal enclave until 1791.

17 Ibid., p. 34.

18 Ibid., pp. 34–5.

19 Ibid., pp. 32–6.

20 Ibid., p. 36.

21 Ibid., p. 37.

22 Brockliss, 'La République des Lettres et les médecins', p. 274.

23 Brockliss, *From Provincial Savant*, pp. 111–389.

24 Ibid., p. 14.

25 Ibid., pp. 188–9. Boulou was the site of a battle in the Pyrenees in 1794 between the French and the First Coalition. Just when Amoreux ceased practising as a physician is unclear.

26 Brockliss, *Calvet's Web*. Les Archives de Société Royale de Médicine list five documents by Calvet.

27 Ibid., pp. 35–6.

28 Whilst Ramel left no record of his income, Calvet averaged 3,114 *livres* per annum over the period 1764–1080. Derived from data in Brockliss, *Calvet's Web*, pp. 29–30.

29 Brockliss, *Calvet's Web*, ch. 5.

30 Brockliss, *From Provincial Savant*, p. 97.

31 Ibid., pp. 54–64.

32 *Annales de La Société Royale de Médicine*, 1786 and 1787/1788; and Brockliss, *From Provincial Savant*, p. 173.
33 Brockliss, *From Provincial Savant*, pp. 54–84.
34 Ibid., p. 55.
35 Ibid., pp. 55–6.
36 Ibid., p. 84.
37 Ibid., p. 89.
38 Ibid., p. 13. See also obituries in the following : Jean-Eugène Dezeimeris, Dictionnaire historique de la médecine ancienne et moderne, ou Précis de l'histoire générale, technologique et littéraire de la médecine; suivi de la Bibliographie médicale du dix-neuvième siècle ; et d'un Répertoire bibliographique par ordre de matières / par MM. Dezeimeris, Ollivier (d'Angers) et Raige-Delorme,...., 4 vols., Paris, Béchet jeune, 1828–39, vol. 3, 1836, pp. 17–18. And, Histoire de la Société royale de médecine..., Avec les Mémoires de médecine et de physique médicale... tirés des registres de cette société, Année 1783. Années 1782 et première partie de 1783, Paris, chez Théophile Barrois le jeune, 1784, pp. 211–16.
39 Collomp, pp. vii, 203–12.
40 Ibid., p. 194.
41 Michel Darluc, *L'histoire naturelle de Provençe* 3 vols., Avignon, Mossey/Niel, 1782–86.
42 *Histoire de la Société royale de médecine*, 1782–83, on Michel Darluc, pp. 210–16.
43 Ibid., vol. 1, pp. 60–70.
44 Brockliss, *From Provincial Savant*, pp. 37–8. *Ecoles centrales* were set up in 1795 to replace the college of art faculties in France's historic universities. They were suppressed in 1802.
45 Ibid., p. 15, and Brockless, *Calvet's Web*, pp. 387–8.

Bibliography

Annales de La Société royale de médicine, 1786 and 1787/1788.

Barthélemy, Louis, *Histoire d'Aubagne: Chef-lieu de baronnie depuis son origine jusq'en 1789*, 2 vols., Marseille, Lafitte reprints, 1972 (Réimpresion de l'édition de Marseille, 1889.).

Brockliss, Laurence W.B., *Calvet's Web: Enlightenment and the Republic of Letters in Eighteenth-Century France*, Oxford, Oxford University Press, 2002.

Brockliss, Laurence W.B., *From Provincial Savant to Parisian Naturalist*, Oxford, Voltaire Foundation, University of Oxford, 2017.

Brockliss, Laurence W.B., 'La République des lettres et les médecins en France à la veille de la Révolution: le cas d'Esprit Calvet', *Gesnerus*, vol. 61, 2004, pp. 254–81.

Brockliss, Laurence and Colin Jones, *The Medical World of Early Modern France*, Oxford, Clarendon Press, 1997.

Collomp, Allain, *Un médecin des lumières: Michel Darluc, naturaliste provençal*, Rennes, Presses universitaires de Rennes, 2011.

Darluc, Michel, *Histoire naturelle de La Provence*, 2 vols., Avignon, chez J.J. Neil, 1782.

Dezeimeris, Jean-Eugène, *Dictionnaire historique de la médecine ancienne et moderne, ou Précis de l'histoire générale, technologique et littéraire de la médecine; suivi de la Bibliographie médicale du dix-neuvième siècle; et d'un Répertoire bibliographique par ordre de matières / par MM. Dezeimeris, Ollivier (d'Angers) et Raige-Delorme,....*, 4 vols., Paris, Béchet jeune, 1828–39.

Histoire de la Société royale de médecine, 1782–83.

10 Conclusions

Ramel did not live a long life, but he experienced the tumult of the Revolution. His family background would have been instrumental in his taking up medicine although his own son did not follow the family tradition. His experiences in North Africa led to his long interest medico-meteorology, which bye-and-large he discounted as an explanation of disease. At various times he maintained a private practice in Aubagne and La Ciotat as well as serving in the hospitals in both of these towns, which would have been the sort of practice one might have expected for a rural doctor. He strove to be a part of the broader medical fraternity as evidenced by his correspondence with the *Société de médicine* and his publications. He was evidently successful; in July 1789 he wrote that the *Sociéte* had awarded him no less than five medals.[1] This was a significant achievement for a country doctor. In terms of the history of medicine, Ramel, despite his efforts to promote himself in as an enlightenment physician, like the majority of his contemporaries, had little impact beyond his own lifetime. His efforts at making a mark on the medicine of the period were largely restricted to France, whereas Amoreux sought international recognition and Calvet focussed on a more local circle of influence.

What drove Ramel to support the revolutionary principles is never clear in his writings. Undoubtedly, he was shocked by the events that took place in his home town, yet he sympathized with the principles that lay behind the changes to French society and ordering of the State brought about by the Revolution. Whether he attached himself to the army in order to escape the excesses he observed in his home region, or, as seems more likely, to make a contribution to the revolutionary cause, can only be conjectured. The *Société royale de médicine* was closed down during the Revolution, along with many other institutions associated with the *ancien régime*, which brought to an end his correspondence with it, though not his book publishing. Reorganization of the teaching of medicine also saw the demise of the Aix medical faculty, which would have disappointed him.

The dominant centres of French medicine in the early-modern period were Paris and Montpellier. Matthew Ramsay, whilst noting it is impossible to know how many physicians there were in eighteenth-century France, suggests that it was at least 2,000–3,000, and possibly more.[2] Whilst many would have been working in Paris and large cities and towns, a significant number must have been working small towns and villages as was the case of Ramel, and Darluc in his early career. Calvet and Amereux on the other hand practised in more substantial towns. This makes Ramel's achievements stand out.

Ramel made considerable effort to make his mark in what he called the Republic of Medicine, and some of his medical writings continued to be referred to long after his death. What light does the biography and writings of this man throw on French medicine and society in the late early-modern period? Many eighteenth-century physicians contested prizes through publications. Ramel's success in this regard was notable, as was the variety of topics he offered to the *Société royale de medicine*. The diagnostic and therapeutic methods he employed were characteristic of his times and accepted by his patients. His interest in medical meteorology was far from unusual although he may have been at odds with many of his contemporaries in concluding the severe limitations of such studies for the advancement of medicine. Equally typical of his times was his condemnation of charlatanism and empiricism. He would not have been the only French physician to have ventured overseas; however, there appears to be no record of meteorological observations by them from French outposts in the period of interest here as Ramel did at La Calle.

Ramel is the only physician I have uncovered from rural France who has left a record of revolutionary fervour. In a letter to Vicq d'Azyr, after the dismemberment of the medical structure of the *ancien régime*, he referred to the "successful revolution", despite how it may have impacted on his own practice and medical practice as a whole.[3] Such discord as was discussed apparently took place in Paris. As has been observed, large numbers of physicians, surgeons, and apothecaries were enlisted into the revolutionary army, but again, these conscripts do not appear to have documented their experiences in war zones.

One cannot avoid thinking that Ramel would have been pleased to know that his work was of interest to historians in the twenty-first century.

Notes

1 Marie-François-Bernadin Ramel, Bibliothéque de l'Académie nationale de médecine, *Archives de la Société royale de médecine (1778–1793)*, Ramel, SRM 180A. fol. 27.
2 Matthew Ramsey, *Professional and Popular Medicine in France, 1770–1830: The Social World of Medical Practice*, Cambridge, Cambridge University Press, 1988. p. 58.
3 Archives de la Société royale de médecine (1778–93), Ramel, SRM 180 A, fol. 40.

Bibliography

Ramel, Marie-François-Bernadin, Bibliothéque de l'Académie nationale de médecine, *Archives de la Société royale de médecine (1778–1793)*, Ramel, SRM 180A. fols. 27 and 40.
Ramsey, Matthew, *Professional and Popular Medicine in France, 1770–1830: The Social World of Medical Practice*, Cambridge, Cambridge University Press, 1988.

Index

Note: Page numbers followed by "n" denote endnotes.

Milton Keynes UK
Ingram Content Group UK Ltd.
UKHW031534071024
449327UK00005B/49